Keto Diet Cookbook for Beginners:

1500 Days of Quick & Easy Keto Recipes to Boost the Immune System and Balance Hormones.

Bonus: 90-Days Workout Plan for Glutes, Legs, Abs and Pecs

Beatrix Sauer & Anna Martin

TABLE OF CONTENTS

1

INTRODUCTION

Today, obesity represents one of the leading causes of death worldwide and is considered one of the most serious public health problems not only in industrialized countries, but also in developing countries.

It has been scientifically demonstrated that the application of ketogenic diet protocols with reduced calorie intake (or *Very Low Calorie Ketogenic Diet*) on obese subjects, allows to obtain positive results in terms of weight loss and reduction of cardiovascular risk factors.

For this reason, today the use of ketogenic diets to promote weight loss is recommended by several scientific communities and is validated and suggested in several states as a therapy of first intention for the treatment of obesity associated with cardiovascular risk factors (diabetes mellitus type 2, insulin resistance, dyslipidemia, hypertension).

Ketogenic diets are low-calorie dietary protocols characterized by reduced carbohydrate intake.

The lack of carbohydrates, involves a lowering of blood levels of insulin, in favor of an increase of glucagon. This hormone has a lipolytic action, promoting the catabolism of triglyceride reserves mobilized from white adipose tissue, which are hydrolyzed thanks to lipoprotein-lipase that promote their transformation into free fatty acids and glycerol.

Fatty acids and glycerol are only partially used for energy purposes: in particular, smooth muscle uses about 40% of free fatty acids, while hepatocytes convert about 10% of mobilized glycerol into glucose.

The remaining portion of fatty acids and glycerol, is metabolized at the hepatic level in the cycles of gluconeogenesis and ketogenesis.

Gluconeogenesis leads to the synthesis of glucose from non-glucose substrates and is rapidly triggered in the absence of glucose by the activity of glucagon.

The reduced glucidic intake of low-calorie ketogenic diets is compensated by an intake of proteins with high biological value. In this condition there is a stabilization of glycemia, through the process of hepatic and renal gluconeogenesis.

The latter phenomenon favors a basal secretion of insulin useful to maintain a stable level of blood ketones. Insulin plays in this sense a modulatory role on ketogenesis itself, making impossible the establishment of pathological ketoacidosis. Therefore during ketogenic low-calorie diets the main source of energy is obtained through the catabolism of reserve lipids, thus determining an effective rapid and constant weight loss at the expense of fat mass.

At the same time, lean mass must be preserved through the intake of an adequate protein quota.

In addition, the ketone bodies produced act on the central nervous system leading to an increase in both the sense of satiety, thanks to the reduction of ghrelin levels and also inducing an improvement in mood.

There are several application protocols of low-calorie diets that induce ketosis, which differ essentially in the different percentages of macronutrients and in the ketogenic ratio achievable.

These ketogenic diets originated for the treatment of several diseases associated with central nervous system degeneration such as epilepsy, Alzheimer's disease and Parkinson's disease, but are currently being used successfully for the reduction of body weight and associated complications in patients suffering from severe obesity and overweight.

Low-calorie ketogenic diet is to be considered a diet therapy and therefore must be managed by experienced personnel able to properly select patients and diseases that can benefit from such therapies, such as hypertension, diabetes mellitus type 2 at the beginning, dyslipidemia, metabolic syndrome, osteopathy or severe arthropathy resulting from excessive overweight, severe obesity with and without indication for bariatric surgery.

It is also essential to ensure close clinical monitoring in order to reduce potential side effects.

Generally, the benefits related to this type of eating plan are rapid weight loss in obese or overweight people with insulin resistance, a reduction in blood fatty acid levels, insulin and fasting blood sugar.

This thesis aims to illustrate principles and applications of the ketogenic diet in the treatment of body weight reduction in patients with obesity.

As an example, a clinical case is also presented to illustrate how the application of this therapeutic regimen allows to obtain satisfactory results in terms of reduction of fat mass even in patients with severe motor problems.

2

HISTORY AND EVOLUTION OF THE KETOGENIC DIET

The Bible reports the use of fasting to heal febrile convulsions, giving fasting a purifying action. Physicians in ancient Greece used to treat diseases, such as epilepsy, by adjusting their patients' diets. A treatise in the Hippocratic Corpus dating back to 400 B.C., *De Morbo Sacro*, considers epilepsy a supernatural disease in origin and cure, and proposes dietary therapy to resolve the physical and mental damage.

In a similar assortment, the creator illustrates the case of a man whose epilepsy disappeared rapidly with total abstaining of food and drink.

It was discovered only centuries later that these intuitions were supported by valid scientific bases. In fact, during prolonged fasting the body enters ketosis, that is, it produces ketone bodies (ketones) which are the basis of the benefits found in the treatments.

Ketones were then discovered in the mid-nineteenth century in the urine of diabetic patients and were considered abnormal products of an incomplete oxidation of fats and therefore considered the cause of the characteristic and devastating clinical picture of diabetic ketoacidosis.

Later in 1822 Radcliffe found an anticonvulsant effect from a diet rich in fat and low in carbohydrates (4:1 ratio).

The main present-day investigation of fasting as a treatment for epilepsy was done in France in 1911. Twenty epileptic patients of any age profited from the constructive outcomes instigated by a low-calorie vegan diet, joined with times of fasting.

The diet led to improvement in the patients' mental abilities, in contrast to their medication, potassium bromide, which clouded the mind.

Also in those years, Dr. Bernarr Macfadden, an American example of actual culture, popularised the use of fasting in order to restore well-being. His disciple, osteopathic physician Hugh Conklin, of Battle Creek, Michigan, began treating his epileptic patients by recommending fasting.

In 1916, Dr. McMurray reported in the New York Medical Journal that he had victoriously examined patients with epilepsy, then followed by a starch- and sugar-free diet, from 1912.

In 1921, endocrinologist H. Rawle Geyelin reported his experiences at the convention of the American Medical Association. He had seen Conklin's prosperity firsthand and had endeavored to recreate the outcomes in 36 of his own patients. He obtained similar results even though having studied the patients for a brief period. Further examinations over the 1920s showed that seizures for the most part relapsed in the wake of fasting. Charles Howland, father of one of Conklin's rewarding patients and a rich New York lawyer, gave his sibling John 5,000 bucks to review "starvation ketosis."

As a teacher of pediatrics at Johns Hopkins Hospital, John Howland utilized the cash to subsidize research led by nervous system specialist Stanley Cobb and his right-hand William G. Lennox.

Beginning in the 1930s, studies of the physiology of ketogenesis and ketolysis established that ketone bodies are physiologically produced in the liver and rapidly utilized by extrahepatic tissues.

Studies were then performed in laboratory animals that demonstrated that injection of β-hydroxybutyrate (BHB) resulted in an increase in its utilization by extrahepatic tissues that correlated with an increase in its blood concentration.

However, once a certain concentration was reached, utilization decreased until BHB accumulated in the blood.

These observations demonstrated that hyperketonemia is achieved only when the ketone bodies produced in the liver exceed the demands of extrahepatic tissues.

In parallel with biochemical researches on the use of ketone bodies by the organism, in the early 20s, studies and investigations on a new dietary regimen involving a reduced intake of carbohydrates (ketogenic diet) were started with the evaluation of its effects on childhood epilepsy. Dr. Russel Wilder and Dr. Peterman of the Mayo Clinic theorized the characteristics of the diet and published the first scientific data related to its experimentation in 1924. (6,11)

Wilder wished to realize to accomplish the advantages of fasting in a dietary treatment that could be kept up with endlessly. His investigation of some epileptic patients in 1921 was the primary utilization of the ketogenic diet as a treatment for epilepsy.

Wilder's colleague, pediatrician Mynie Peterman, later formulated the classic diet (KD), with a ratio of one gram of protein per kilogram of body weight in children, 10-15 gr of carbohydrates per day, and the rest of the calories from fat. Peterman's work over the 20s has established techniques for inducing and maintaining a state of ketosis in the diet. Peterman archived constructive outcomes (further developed wakefulness, conduct, and rest) and negative outcomes (sickness and nausea because of overabundance ketosis). The diet proved to be very effective in children: in 1925 Peterman reported that 95% of 37 young patients had improved and in 60% of cases the disease had regressed.

By 1930, diet was additionally applied in 100 young people and grown-ups. Although the results in adults were similar to modern results in children, they did not compare with contemporary studies. Barborka presumed that grown-ups would be more averse to profit from the eating routine, and the utilization of the ketogenic diet in grown-ups was not examined again until 1999.

In 1958, a study conducted by Richard E. Johnson and his research group on a sample of 208 healthy young people given a normal diet and moderate physical activity showed that serum and urine always had measurable levels of ketones. The concentration Johnson found was about 0.7mM/L, about 20 times as low as the levels found in patients with untreated type I diabetes mellitus.

In 1966 George F. Cahill and his group were able to put together a series of useful observations to explain the importance of ketone bodies as an emergency fuel for various organs and body systems (13,14).

In 1971, after extensive studies, Prof. Blackburn of Harvard University in the United States outlined the protocol of the *Protein Sparing Modified Fasting* diet (Lidner and Blackburn 1976) for the treatment of obesity. (15,16)

In 1972 Dr. Atkins published a book where he outlined a ketogenic low-calorie, but high-protein dietary protocol to achieve an effective weight loss.

In 1975, Professor Marineau, a student of Blackburn, defined the protocol as "Jeune proteinè" (protein fasting) for a distinction between the Blackburn method and Atkins-type high-protein diets (Marineau 2004).

In the 90s, the *Very Low Calorie Ketogenic Diet* protocol was adopted at John Hopkins Hospital in Baltimore.

In 1993, the U.S. Department of Health through a task force (JAMA), validates the protocol of the low calorie ketogenic diet.

In 1995, Richard L. Veech and his research group were able to demonstrate how ketone bodies could be useful in compensating for dysfunction due to insulin resistance, thus opening up a whole series of new opportunities for the therapeutic use of ketogenic diets.

In 1997, Professor Björntorp deepens the study of the protocol of low calorie ketogenic diet, publishing the result of his research in the journal Lancet.

Since 2000, the attention towards the use of ketogenic diets increases and a series of works that analyze the potential therapeutic uses of ketogenic diets in the treatment of degenerative diseases of the CNS (such as Alzheimer's, Parkinson's, epilepsy) and metabolic diseases such as insulin resistance and obesity begin to appear.

In 2003, the Finnish Ministry of Health suggested the low-calorie ketogenic diet as a therapy of first intention for the treatment of obesity associated with cardiovascular risk factors (type 2 diabetes mellitus, insulin resistance, dyslipidemia, hypertension).

The ADI, Association of Dietetics and Clinical Nutrition, in 2014 proposed the Ketogenic Diet as a therapy for obesity, as well as for a number of other metabolic-based diseases.

In the same year, Dr. Moreno and his associates outline in a key article the short- and long term benefits obtained from the low-calorie ketogenic diet compared with the classic reduced-calorie diet (LCD).

3

BIOCHEMICAL PRINCIPLES OF THE KETOGENIC DIET: KETOSIS

Ketone bodies

The ketogenic diet is based on a drastic reduction of carbohydrates, combined with a relative increase in the share of proteins and fats.

This condition pushes the organism into ketosis, that is a metabolic status characterized by an expansion in the convergence of ketone bodies in the blood.

Ketone bodies are three products of hepatic ketogenesis:

- Acetoacetate (AcAc), which can be converted by the liver into β-hydroxybutyrate, or spontaneously transformed into acetone

- Acetone (Ac), which is generated through the decarboxylation of acetoacetate, either spontaneously or through the enzyme acetoacetate decarboxylase.

- B-hydroxybutyrate (BHB) (not in fact a ketone as per IUPAC classification) is created through the activity of the catalyst D-β-hydroxybutyrate dehydrogenase on acetoacetate.

- B-Hydroxybutyrate is the most bountiful ketone body, trailed by acetoacetate lastly CH3)2CO.

β-Hydroxybutyrate and acetoacetate can undoubtedly go through membranes and are consequently a wellspring of energy for the cerebrum, which can't use unsaturated fats straightforwardly.

The Ketone bodies exhibit general chemical characteristics that regulate their functionality:

- They are acidic compounds (pK-4)

- They are water-soluble metabolites of fatty acids and therefore do not require blood transporters

- Small size and thus are favored in the passage of plasma and hematoencephalic membranes

- Have an insulin-independent uptake

Ketogenesis

Under physiological conditions, oxidative decarboxylation of pyruvic acid and beta-oxidation are regulated so that no acetyl CoA is produced in excess of what the cell can use.

These primarily involve the complete oxidation of acetyl CoA in the mitochondria to CO_2 and H_2O or, in tissues where they occur, the cytosolic utilization of acetyl CoA for the biosynthesis of fatty acids and, to a lesser extent, cholesterol.

Mitochondrial oxidation of acetyl CoA depends on mitochondrial levels of oxaloacetate, which is produced primarily by carboxylation of pyruvic acid, the terminal product of glycolysis and metabolism of certain amino acids (alanine, serine, glycine).

Indeed, acetyl CoA and oxaloacetate condense to form citrate, which is consumed in the mitochondrion in the terminal oxidative pathway (citric acid cycle) or exported to the cytosol (fatty acid and cholesterol biosynthesis).

Therefore, the utilization of acetyl CoA in the mitochondria requires a proper metabolism of amino acids and especially carbohydrates that ensures the cell an adequate supply of pyruvate and therefore of oxaloacetate.

During a ketogenic dietary regimen, characterized by reduced availability of carbohydrates, their energy intake is replaced by that provided by increased fat catabolism.

Under these conditions, gluconeogenesis from pyruvate produced by the metabolism of amino acids is generally favored instead of glycolysis in order to ensure the availability of the minimum amount of glucose necessary for the metabolism of nerve cells and erythrocytes.

Therefore, an imbalance is determined between the production of pyruvate and oxaloacetate (whose levels also decrease due to their utilization in gluconeogenesis) and that of acetyl CoA (whose levels increase due to increased metabolic utilization of fatty acids), in favor of the latter.

In liver cells, excess acetyl CoA in the mitochondria is partly converted into ketone bodies: acetoacetate, β-hydroxybutyrate, and acetone, which accumulate in the blood and are either used by other tissues or eliminated in the urine.

Mitochondrial synthesis of ketone bodies occurs in three steps: reaction of two acetyl CoA molecules to form acetoacetyl CoA

1. reaction of acetoacetyl CoA with a third acetyl CoA molecule to form 3-hydroxy-3-methyl-glutaryl-CoA (HMG-CoA)

2. split of HMG-CoA into acetoacetate and acetyl CoA

Acetoacetate, the main ketone body, is partly reduced to BHB or decarboxylated to acetone, a volatile substance eliminated by respiration, urine, and sweat.

Liver cells spill acetoacetate and BHB into the circulation, which are taken up by cells in peripheral tissues, particularly myocardium, skeletal muscle, and brain.

Metabolic fate of ketone bodies

Ketone bodies are used by extrahepatic target organs primarily as fuels, producing 2 molecules of GTP and 22 ATP per molecule of acetoacetate when oxidized in mitochondria.

Energy utilization of acetoacetate requires its activation to acetoacetyl CoA by reaction with succinyl CoA, an intermediate in the citric acid cycle; then acetoacetyl CoA is split into two acetyl CoA molecules to produce reducing equivalents (NADH and FADH2), in a reaction identical to the last reaction of fatty acid beta-oxidation. These reactions are catalyzed by the enzyme β-ketoacyl-CoA transferase, likewise called thioporase, which is absent in the liver.

Acetone in low concentrations is absorbed by the liver and undergoes detoxification through the methylcyloxy pathway ending in lactate.

Acetone in high concentrations is taken up by cells other than the liver and enters a pathway that converts 1,2-propanediol to pyruvate with ATP consumption.

The heart preferentially uses fatty acids as fuel under normal physiological conditions. However, under conditions of ketosis, it can actually use ketones for this purpose.

Under conditions of prolonged fasting, the brain can also use as fuel ketone bodies, which, unlike fatty acids, can cross the blood-brain barrier.

As glucose and ketone bodies have a comparative KM (Michaelis-Menten consistent) for the transportation of glucose in the mind, ketone bodies begin to be utilized in the CNS when they arrive at a worth of around 4 mM, which is that of the monocarboxylase carrier.

The ketone bodies in addition to being used by the body in the production of energy, also perform the following functions:

- Increase the antioxidant capacity of the cell up to 50%, decreasing by about 55% the reactive oxygen species (ROS).

- They elevate gamma-butyric acid (GABA) levels while inhibiting the transmission of glutaminergic signals.

- Increase up to 4 times glutathione peroxidase activity in the hippocampus

- They uncouple cytochrome oxidase and cause shifts in heat production to ATP production through increased UCP protein levels.

- Increases sodium/potassium pumps in both neurons and glia cells, increasing membrane potential and decreasing excitability

- They inhibit phosphofructokinase by reducing the rate of glycolysis and free radical production, while increasing the substrates available for energy production in the Krebs cycle (anaplerotic reaction)

- They affect mediators responsible for detecting the energy status of cells (PPAR, mTOR, sirtuins) and thus promote the maintenance of cellular energy homeostasis

- They act as cellular signals responsible for the inhibition of histone deacetylases (HDACs) and make chromatin more easily readable to transcriptase. They therefore interact with gene expression

- Modulate mechanisms of cell aging and death

Hematochemical parameters under ketosis conditions

Because they are produced by hepatic metabolism, ketones are normally present in the blood, albeit in low amounts, and their concentration is referred to as ketonemia.

Under normal conditions, ketonemia does not exceed 0,5 mmol/L.

The concentration of free AcAc in physiological conditions is therefore negligible and once produced it is transported into the circulation and easily metabolized in various tissues and in particular in skeletal muscle and heart.

Under conditions of overproduction, however, acetoacetic acid accumulates and some of it is transformed into the other two ketone bodies (BHB and Ac).

The presence of ketone bodies in the flow and their disposal in the urine cause ketonemia and ketonuria.

The elimination of acetone, being an extremely unstable compound, occurs mostly by pulmonary breathing and sweating.

In ketoacidosis, the blood (or urinary) concentration of AcAc and BHB can be measured and the lactate/pyruvate ratio assessed.

The dual measurement of the Lactate/Pyruvate and BHB/AcAc ratio is an index of the body's redox state related to the NAD+/NADH ratio.

The BHB assay is used more than the AcAc assay; and the ratio of ketone bodies gives information of great value in the evaluation

metabolic.

The normal ratio BHB / AcAc is 3:1 but in ketosis there are also values of 6:1 and up to 12:1.

In physiological ketosis (which is reached during fasting and ketogenic diets) ketonemia reaches maximum levels of 7/8 mM with an unchanged pH, while in decompensated diabetes it reaches and exceeds 20 mM with a lowering of the pH.

The blood values of ketone bodies do not exceed, in a healthy individual, the 8 mM because the CNS efficiently uses these molecules for energy purposes in place of glucose.

Furthermore, in physiological ketosis, blood glucose, although lowering, remains at physiological levels. In fact, glucose formed from gluconeogenic amino acids and glycerol released from triglyceride lysis is sufficient for the maintenance of euglycemia.

Figure 1shows a summary diagram of the main blood values found under physiological conditions, under ketosis and under ketoacidosis.

Blood values	Normal Diet	Ketogenic Diet	Diabetic keto-acidosis
Glucose (mg/dL)	80–120	65–80	>300
Insulin (µU/L)	6–23	6,6–9,4	=0
DC Concentration(mM/L)	0,1	7/8	>25
pH	7,4	7,4	<7,3

Figure 1 Blood values of some reference parameters during a normal, ketogenic diet and during diabetic ketoacidosis

KETOGENIC DIETARY PROTOCOLS

There are several ketogenic dietary protocols that differ from each other based on calories, percentages of different macronutrients, and the achievable ketogenic ratio.

The term ketogenic ratio refers to the ratio (R) between the amount of lipids in grams present in the dietary protocol and the amount of protein and carbohydrates.

The main ketogenic dietary therapies that are used to treat CNS diseases in the clinical setting are:

- The Classic Ketogenic Diet (KD)

- The ketogenic medium-chain triglyceride diet (MCT)

    The ketogenic dietary regimes that are instead mainly used for the treatment of obesity, as they exploit ketosis and caloric reduction to obtain a rapid and constant loss of fat mass, are:

- Modified Atkins Diet (MAD)

- Low Glycemic Index Ketogenic Diet (LGIT)

- Fat-fasting

- Very low calorie ketogenic diet

Classic Ketogenic Diet (KD)

The classic ketogenic diet (KD) was introduced in 1920 to try to mimic the ketosis resulting from fasting, since the latter had been shown to be effective in treating seizures that were not pharmaceutically treatable.

Classic KD was first used at the Mayo Clinic and later revived at the Johns Hopkins University Medical Center neurology clinic.

The KD protocol remains the most effective anti-convulsive dietary protocol ever and is the gold standard.

This diet contains a ketogenic ratio of 4:1. This means that for every total gram of protein plus carbohydrates contained in the diet there must be grams4 of lipids.

This is achieved by barring high-carb food varieties like products of the soil, breads, pastas, grains, and sugar, while expanding utilization of high-fat food varieties like nuts, cream, and margarine.

Most dietary fats are long-chain fatty substances (LCT). This kind of convention has the accompanying detriments:

- Is too strict and no non-prescribed meals or snacks are permitted

- It is unbalanced

- Could be harmful to the intestinal microbiota

- The use of lipid, mineral and vitamin supplements is required.

- Poor patient adherence to the protocol because it is too restrictive

- High drop out.

Medium-Chain Triglyceride (MCT) Diet

A variant to KD is MCT. This protocol was developed by Huttenlocher and collaborators in the Department of Paediatrics at University of Yale.

It is a diet rich in medium-chain triglycerides (MCTs) that allow to maintain a high ketogenic ratio (3:1) even in the presence of greater amounts of carbohydrates and proteins, since the oxidation of MCTs results in greater production of ketones than the long-chain triglycerides used in KD.

In addition, MCTs are better absorbed than long-chain triglycerides and are transported to the liver by portal vein blood flow.

The MCT diet contains about 60% fat and can lead to troublesome intestinal disorders. For this reason, a variant of this protocol has been developed that involves reducing the MCT fat portion to 30% (modified MCT).

Modified MCT has the advantage of not resulting in gastrointestinal symptoms, although it may make it more difficult to maintain ketosis at the 3:1 ratio.

In the MCT diet, MCT oil is used as the lipid source.

The oil is blended in with no less than two times its volume of skim milk, chilled, tasted during a supper or integrated into food.

However, frequent side effects in this type of dietary protocol bring a high drop out.

The MCT diet has replaced KD in many hospitals, although some diets are designed as a combination of the two.

Modified Atkins Diet (MAD)

The MAD protocol (modified Atkins Diet) is a dietary protocol designed in 2003 to mimic the high-fat KD diet by allowing greater introduction of protein, lipids, and calories to increase compliance, especially in adult patients. (28,29) The MAD is a modified model of the diet devised in 1970s by Robert Coleman Atkins, an American cardiologist who was the first physician to hypothesize the utility and sustainability of a low-carbohydrate nutritional regimen for the prevention of metabolic disease.

Dr. Atkins proposed this type of diet for the treatment of overweight and obesity and related diseases believing that the cause of the obesity that was spreading in the United States was attributable to the excessively high carbohydrate diet (1963). He was also the first to link obesity to a state of hyperinsulinemia and developed his own protocol to treat his severely overweight condition.

His diet was a very effective slimming regimen and it spread very quickly. However he became the target of a series of criticisms which were based on the fact that the assumptions of his theory were wrong as the increase of insulin levels were to be considered a consequence of obesity and not its cause.

His other criticism was that the excessive fat intake within his diet could increase his risk of cardiovascular disease.

After his death, the scientific theories postulated by Atkins regarding hyperinsulinemia were confirmed by other scientists and scientifically explained through insulin resistance.

Currently, MAD is the most widely used ketogenic protocol when deciding to apply ketosis to the treatment of obesity.

The ketogenic ratio of MAD is significantly lower than previous ketogenic protocols (0.9-1:1).

In fact, it requires that only 65% of the nutrients in the diet derive from lipids (as opposed to 90% in KD) and makes the structuring of meals much simpler. The implementation of MAD as described in the protocols of John Hopkins University is based on several steps that lead to the induction of a state of ketosis and then maintain it with the lowest possible level of ketonemia.

It is based on carbohydrate restriction, initially 10 gr/day in children and 15 gr/day in adults; dose that is increased to 20-30 gr/day after a couple of months.

Any type of carbohydrate is allowed on the menu, and the amount of carbohydrate can be divided into different meals or taken all at once, and fiber is not counted as carbohydrate.

As with KD, MAD also requires supplementation of certain vitamins and minerals.

Low Glycemic Index Ketogenic Diet (LGIT)

LGIT (low glycemic index treatment) is a treatment protocol based on the choice of low glycemic index (GI) foods.

The GI is a measure of the increase in circulating glucose levels in response to ingestion of a specific food. The index estimates how each gram of carbohydrate available in a food source will increase blood glucose levels compared to consumption of pure glucose, which is assigned a GI of 100.

The GI therefore measures the glycemic power of a carbohydrate, that is the ability to release a certain amount of glucose after digestion.

The LGIT diet is a ketogenic nutritional strategy that aims to achieve extremely stable glycemic levels, but with a less restrictive approach than other ketogenic diets.

The carbohydrates allowed in the LGIT diet are limited to those that have a GI < 50, as the theoretical hypothesis underlying this dietary protocol is that maintaining of a stably low blood glucose level is one of the reasons for the effectiveness of ketogenic diets.

Total caloric intake is determined according to the patient's needs, with 20-30% of calories coming from protein and the remaining 60% from fat, and with a higher carbohydrate intake than KD, MCT, and MAD diets (40-60 gr/day).

However, the proportion of carbohydrates in the diet is low, as it represents about 10% of the total macronutrients (lower than in MCT protocols).

Although carbohydrates remain low, the high protein quota (about 30%) means that LGIT achieves a low ketogenic ratio (0.6:1), thus a lower ketonemia than can be obtained with other diets.

There are numerous studies in the literature that propose LGIT as a dietary plan of excellence in the treatment of childhood obesity and it has also been successfully tested in the treatment of diabetic patients (reduction of glucose levels, insulin, glycated hemoglobin and fructosamine).

Fat-fasting or ketogenic fasting

This is an integration between a fasting or semi-fasting phase and a ketogenic diet phase.

The calorie restriction (CR) and the intermittent fasting (IF) have been displayed to apply the same effects at both metabolic and cellular levels.

Thus, this dietary protocol is designed to achieve higher ketonemia levels and increase the effects of the ketogenic diet.

Intermittent fasting (IF) is a nutritional strategy based on a cyclized diet that, although not necessarily involving a reduction of calories, allows to obtain the same results of a low-calorie diet in terms of neuroprotection, cardioprotection, increased insulin sensitivity and selective cell apoptosis.

There are a variety of intermittent fasting protocols ranging from 24-hour fasting, to calorie reduction every other day, to reducing the hourly window in which you feed.

These protocols are often combined with ketogenic dietary regimens to increase ketonemia levels.

The resulting diet will be a mix of CR/IF and the chosen ketogenic regimen, and will therefore be defined as fat-fasting or ketogenic fasting.

It is a highly unbalanced regimen and must be implemented for short periods (a few days) for example to accelerate the state of induction of ketosis.

This dietary therapy should be done under close medical monitoring.

In cases of patients following a ketogenic regimen for the treatment of obesity, the fat-fasting protocol can be used with greater freedom. For example, two days per week can be provided in cases of obesity treatment in which the MAD followed by patients can be modified with calorie restriction (CR).

In fact, this treatment is broadly utilized in the treatment of obesity to increment weight reduction.

The difference between fat-fast and fat-fasting is that while the former protocol involves strong caloric restriction, the latter can also be isocaloric and for this reason can be followed for longer.

Ketogenic reduced calorie diets

Modern very low calorie ketogenic diets are based on the principles of the Blackburn diet (Lidner et al. 1976) and are characterized by:

- A low calorie content (<800 Cal/day)

- The development of a stable and controlled ketosis

- Selective reduction of fat mass

They contemplate a reduced total intake of carbohydrates (between 0.5 and 0.9 gr/kg body weight, to trigger and maintain a state of ketosis) and lipids (0.2-0.5 gr/kg body weight, enough to prevent cholelithiasis), while including a physiological amount of proteins (1.2 ± 0.2 gr/kg body weight) as well as a balanced intake of vegetable fibers, water, vitamins, minerals and trace elements.

Unsweetened liquids (>2 liters/day) and cooked and raw vegetables promote the hydration of lean mass, tissue elasticity, protein synthesis, and counteract constipation, hyperazotemia, hyperuricemia and kidney stones; they are associated with meal replacements containing proteins of high biological value derived mainly from legumes and milk with a standardized intake of essential nutrients.

This slimming phase, in order to stabilize the weight result, is followed by a transition phase, whose duration is at least equal to that of slimming and which is divided into 4 stages in which both the quantity and the quality of carbohydrate foods with a low index and glycemic load are gradually increased, until reaching the maintenance phase, characterized by a balanced, normocaloric Mediterranean-type diet.

Contraction of dietary carbohydrate intake reduces the insulin/glucagon ratio, which induces ketosis as early as 48-72 hours.

These low-calorie diets allow to significantly reduce blood pressure and lipid values, already after 24-48 hours and contribute, in the medium and long term, to decrease the cardiometabolic and oncological risk related to diabetes and visceral obesity.

5

OBESITY AND KETOGENIC DIETS

Although ketogenic diets originated as a dietary/therapeutic treatment of epilepsy and have demonstrated scientifically proven positive effects in many diseases (Polycystic Ovary Syndrome (PCOS), acne, cluster headaches, neurodegenerative diseases and cancer), the area in which they are of greatest interest today is in the treatment of obesity and related risk factors.

The focus on the application of low-calorie ketogenic dietary therapies in the treatment of obesity has recently been brought to the forefront within the international scientific community thanks to a study by Dr. Moreno B. and a group of researchers that emphasizes the long-term benefits of a reduced-calorie ketogenic diet over a diet that simply involves calorie restriction.

Also in Italy, in 2014, the ADI, Association of Dietetics and Clinical Nutrition, has expressed its support for the use of the ketogenic diet as a therapy for obesity, as well as for a number of other metabolic-based diseases.

Currently, low-calorie ketogenic dietary therapies find wide application in patients with severe obesity who do not respond to other types of low-calorie diets or who do not have the ability to engage in regular physical activity.

Obesity

Obesity is a chronic condition, characterized by an excessive increase in adipose tissue with repercussions on the state of health.

It is caused much of the time by erroneous ways of life: from one viewpoint, a mistaken hypercaloric diet and on the other a decreased energy consumption because of actual dormancy. Obesity represents one of the really general medical conditions overall both on the grounds that its pervasiveness is continually expanding in Western nations as well as in mid-low pay nations and in light of the fact that it is a significant gamble factor for different constant sicknesses, for example, type 2 diabetes mellitus, cardiovascular illnesses and cancers. It is assessed that 44% of type 2 diabetes cases, 23% of ischemic coronary illness cases, and up to 41% of certain tumors are owing to obesity/overweight. Altogether, overweight and stoutness imply the fifth most significant danger factor for worldwide mortality, and passings owing to heftiness are no less than 2.8 million/year around the world.

The body mass index (BMI) or according to the more commonly used acronym BMI (Weight record Index), is a value (biometric data) that compares weight and height, allowing to evaluate if a person is normal weight (BMI: 18.50 - 24.99), underweight (BMI < 18.50), overweight (25-30) or obese (BMI =/> 30).

The percentage of the population in excess weight increases as age increases and, in particular, overweight goes from 14% in the 18-24 age group to 46% between 65-74 years, while obesity goes from 2.3% to 15.3% for the same age groups. Moreover, the condition of excess weight is more widespread among men than women (overweight: 44% vs 27.3%; obesity: 10.8% vs 9%).

In Europe, the weight record has a typical worth of 26.5. Between 30 and 70% of the adult population are overweight, while 10-30% of people are obese (about 20% of men and 23% of women) (World Health organization - Europe, 2008).

As indicated by WHO information, the commonness of obesity around the world multiplied from 1980 to 2014.

In the meantime, the problem has now begun to affect younger segments of the population as well: in 2011, it is estimated that there were more than 40 million overweight children under the age of 5 in the world.

"The Moreno Study": Efficacy of the low-calorie ketogenic diet in the treatment of obesity

Many controlled studies show that ketogenic diets are effective in promoting significant weight loss in all treated subjects, while improving the main metabolic risk indices associated with overweight and obesity.

Ketogenic low-calorie diets in fact allow you to:

- Lower insulin levels

- Decrease the signal effect of IGFs

- Induce the production of FoxO

- Stimulate AMP-activated protein kinases (AMPK)

- Repress mTOR protein

- Promote the transcription of genes that increase the production of antioxidants

All these metabolic effects increase weight loss by improving glycemic tolerance, insulin resistance, so that in some cases may be an excellent dietary therapy for type 2 diabetes.

In 2014, a review directed by Dr. Moreno B. highlighted the results of using the low-calorie ketogenic diet.

This study, for the first time in the literature, focuses on the long-term effects of a ketogenic hypocaloric diet, demonstrating that it is effective in the treatment of obesity not only in the first months but also and especially in the years following the end of the therapy itself.

Moreno demonstrates not only that low-calorie ketogenic diet therapy is more effective than low-calorie diet therapy (LCD) in the 12 months after completion, but also in the 24 months in both anthropometric and commorbidity terms.

The study included 45 obese subjects (BMI≥30) with a clinical history of repeated dieting and poor outcomes.

In accordance with European guidelines, all selected subjects did not present type I diabetes mellitus, endocrinological or medications disorders, were not depressed or with mental problems, dependent on drugs or medications, with severe renal failure, with gout, with previous cardiovascular episodes or cerebrovascular disorders, uncontrolled hypertension, electrolyte alterations, pregnant or lactating. Furthermore, subjects treated with other forms of diets with anti-obesity drugs in the 6 months preceding the start of ketogenic treatment were excluded.

Subjects involved in the study were randomized into two groups: one treated with the low-calorie ketogenic diet, the other with an LCD. The control group (LCD) followed a 1400- 1800 Kcal diet consisting of 15-25% protein, 45-55% carbohydrate, 25-35% lipids, and 20/40 gr/day of fiber.

The therapy with the ketogenic low-calorie diet included 3 phases: the active ketogenic phase (600-800 Kcal) using commercial products rich in proteins with high biological value and low in lipids and carbohydrates (<50 gr of carbohydrates per day, 0.8 gr of protein/1,2 kg of ideal weight), a phase of dietary re-education with gradual re-introduction of carbohydrates and lipids, and a phase of weight maintenance achieved through a balanced diet of 1500-2000 Kcal.

Moreno and his associates have shown that from the start of dietary therapy until two years after completion, weight loss is twice as great when treated with a low-calorie ketogenic diet compared to an LCD.

Consistently, the reduction of different anthropometric parameters is significantly greater in subjects treated with a low-calorie ketogenic diet.

The analysis of body composition shows that lean mass remains constant both during the dietary treatment and in the two years following the end of the same, while fat mass tends to return to initial levels, although remaining significantly lower in patients treated with a ketogenic hypocaloric diet (8.8 kg for the low-calorie ketogenic diet vs 3.8 kg in the LCD, $p<0.001$).

Furthermore, by analyzing the location of fat mass lost, the low-calorie ketogenic diet is selective on visceral fat.

Finally, the study demonstrates that the low-calorie ketogenic diet is more effective in maintaining long-term weight loss. Two years after the end of the diet, 54% of subjects treated with a low-calorie ketogenic diet maintained a weight loss greater than 10% of their initial weight, while with LCD only 13% (p<0.001).

In addition, diet therapy low-calorie ketogenic diet allows to delay the recovery of lost weight, thus the reappearance of the disease and commorbidities.

Advantages and contraindications of the ketogenic diet

The ketogenic diet has numerous advantages in the treatment of obesity and other diseases, however, it has limitations and contraindications.

Benefits include:

- The motivational factor related to the rapid activation of weight loss;

- The reduction in hunger associated with moderate ketosis;

- A better maintenance of trophism and muscle mass;

- A better adherence to the diet experienced by the patient as a personalized therapy

Possible benefits related to the fact that these therapies can be applied in risk groups for preventive purposes are also reported in the literature.

Several papers also report ketogenic diets as a valuable support to bariatric surgery, e.g. facilitating a preoperative decline in order to reduce generic risk and post-surgical complications, improving comorbidities associated with severe obesity.

However, ketogenic dietary protocols that are high in fat (little used in body weight reduction treatment) could, if not structured properly, increase lipemic risk indicators that are commonly associated with obesity.

Another side effect of ketogenic diets concerns the risk of kidney damage, since obese people often already have a decrease in the number of functioning nephrons, which is often associated with high blood pressure.

In addition, obese individuals often have diabetic comorbidity, which can lead to additional renal function issues.

However, it has been shown that in subjects undergoing studies, these risks turn out to be potential and that a ketogenic diet is even able to reverse experimentally induced diabetic nephropathy in an animal model.

Another potential risk, due to both diet-induced ketosis and the subject's state of obesity, is bone demineralization.

However, subjects are not treatable with ketogenic low-calorie diets if they're suffering from:

- Type I diabetes mellitus

- Severe liver failure (chronic active hepatitis, cirrhosis)

- Renal insufficiency and GF <60 ml/min or creatinineemia higher than 1,5 mg/dl

- Serious cardiac pathologies: heart failure, atrio-ventricular conduction blocks, arrhythmic pathology

- Myocardial infarction and stroke occurred in the 3 months preceding the beginning of the dietary treatment

- Serious psychiatric illness, drug or alcohol abuse

- Treatment with non-potassium-sparing diuretics and unbalanced hypokalaemia

- Chronic systemic therapy with corticosteroid medications

- Pregnancy and lactation

Induction of ketosis can lead to different problems in the early days of therapy or later stages.

To improve the therapeutic effect while reducing the risk of side effects, close medical supervision and periodic monitoring of adherence to indications, clinical conditions and any blood chemistry data is necessary.

Headache, the most frequent early side effect present in about one-third of patients, tends to disappear spontaneously within 72 hours.

Halitosis, xerostomia, and constipation are subsequently described. Some patients also report impaired cold tolerance and postural vertigo.

An increased incidence of biliary disorders and cholelithiasis has been reported, sometimes leading to cholecystectomy.

Monitoring a ketogenic diet

Before starting a ketogenic diet, a general evaluation of the patient is necessary, aiming to ascertain:

- Nutritional status

- The basal metabolic rate

- Any metabolic abnormalities

- The state of bone mineralization

- Renal function

- Neurological status

This investigation should also be combined with an abdominal ultrasound and screening for any contraindications, aimed at preventing catabolic seizures, proceeding to dosing:

- Plasma levels of lactic and pyruvic acid

- Plasma and urinary amino acid levels

- Urinary organic acid levels

- Of plasma carnitine and acylcarnitine levels

Another useful investigation is the gut microbiome test.

Once all parameters are verified to be within limits, proceed to start the diet gradually (if it has a high ketogenic ratio).

Ketosis is usually monitored using blood or urine.

Strips for urinary ketone analysis can be used for self-testing. It is important to remember that once opened they have a shelf life of two months and are inactivated by humidity and temperatures above 30°C.

6

APPLICATION OF KETOGENIC DIETARY PROTOCOLS IN THE TREATMENT OF OBESITY

In the following paragraph we will detail, as an example, a ketogenic diet therapy applied to the treatment of obesity: MAD with natural foods.

Example of a MAD protocol for the treatment of obesity

The MAD ketogenic dietary protocol used for weight loss is a hypoglucidic and hyperlipidic diet.

The effectiveness in fast and steady slimming is favored:

- By a reduced intake of carbohydrates that favors the state of ketosis

- By the sense of satiety due to the release of cholecystokinin

- By the production of anabolic hormones (such as testosterone and growth hormone) that increase lean mass and improve metabolic function.

The MAD diet program has four stages, balancing, induction, pre-maintenance and maintenance.

PHASE 1: INDUCTION OR APPROACH TO THE DIET

During the induction phase, which lasts at least 2 weeks during which the body must get used to the new rhythm, you can introduce a maximum of 15 grams of glucose per day, eliminating complex carbohydrates such as pasta, bread, rice, cereals, potatoes, sugary drinks, and some fruits and vegetables, while you can take without limitation fatty foods and proteins such as eggs, red meat, cheese, and some types of vegetables.

The use of foods with high lipid content is strongly recommended.

This stage trains the body to consume fat appropriately and keep glucose levels constant.

PHASE 2: BALANCING

In the second balancing phase, the same type of diet is maintained only that about 5 gr of extra glucose per day is gradually introduced. We proceed with the intake of non-sugary fresh fruits and nuts, until we reach the so-called "critical carbohydrate level" that the body needs to reduce its weight. It is planned to reach 25 gr of carbohydrates in the week in which you started this second phase of the diet, 30grr in the following week until our weight loss comes to a halt.

The duration of this phase is variable as it is linked to the rate at which you lose weight which is different from person to person.

PHASE 3: PRE-MAINTENANCE

In the third phase, pre-maintenance, the amount of glucose is increased by about 10 grams per week, and weight loss is reduced to about 500 grams per week. The intake of carbohydrates is established through the intake of foods such as yogurt and fruit, including sugary ones (always paying attention to quantities).

STEP 4: MAINTENANCE.

The maintenance phase consists of taking the maximum amount of carbohydrates that, through the phases of the diet, has come to define as "critical level of carbohydrates for weight maintenance", that is, that amount of carbohydrates to provide the body with glucose essential for some of the vital processes. In general, however, this quantity never exceeds 90 grams of glucose per day.

In MAD, the use of specific supplements is expected: antioxidants, multivitamins and fiber-based.

Antioxidant supplements are useful because, being a diet rich in animal fats (meat and fish) and polyunsaturated fats (fish and nuts) that produce an increased diffusion and action of free radicals, help to prevent premature aging, oxidative stress and degenerative diseases.

Among the antioxidant supplements you can choose those based on: vitamin A; vitamin C; vitamin E; selenium; zinc; copper; caffeic acid; blueberries; berries; green tea; ginko biloba; rose hips; wheat germ oil.

Multivitamin supplements are very important because of the dietary restrictions of such a diet (the intake of fruits and grains is greatly reduced).

In the MAD diet, the reduced consumption of grains and fruits deprives some of the fiber intake, so the use of fiber supplements is recommended.

Fiber plays an important role as it improves the functionality of the intestine and reduces the risk of contracting degenerative diseases, cardiovascular diseases, diabetes and some types of cancer such as colorectal cancer.

Fiber supplements include those made from: guar gum, karaya gum, psyllium, pectin, glucomannan and bran.

Below is a list of disadvantages associated with MAD dietic therapy:

- This is a highly unbalanced diet (fat 65%, ketogenic ratio about 1)

- Diseases such as osteoporosis and gout can occur due to excessive calciuria, which also induces the formation of kidney stones;

- Must be associated with high fluid consumption to avoid body dehydration

- Problems such as constipation due to lack of fiber or diarrhea (in the induction phase) may occur

- Insomnia

- Nausea, vomiting, hypotension, increased respiratory rate

- Halitosis.

The MAD diet should be considered diet therapy and therefore should be managed by experienced staff.

7

SUMMING UP

The use of ketogenic dietary therapies is now recommended by several scientific communities in the treatment of obesity and other related conditions.

Data in the literature show that the ketogenic diet is a valuable support in weight reduction in individuals with obesity.

Ketogenic dietary protocols, properly prepared and supervised by competent personnel, are used to treat patients with severe obesity, in whom the application of other dietary therapies has not brought satisfactory results.

The main cause of failure of classic hypocaloric diets is to be found in most cases in the inability of the patient to carry out physical activity (patients who are bedridden or with disabling diseases) and therefore to consume glucidic and lipidic reserves in an appropriate way.

The state of ketosis, which is established in patients undergoing ketogenic dietary therapy, allows instead to activate metabolic pathways with high lipid consumption and therefore to obtain better results in the short and long term.

In fact, many studies confirm the short- and long-term benefits of this type of diet compared to low-calorie diets with normal carbohydrate content or diets with reduced lipid intake.

However, there is insufficient data to attest to the clear superiority of one dietary regimen over another in terms of long-term benefits and safety.

The use of ketogenic diets has in fact contraindications and disadvantages that must be properly evaluated before their application. Being a diet therapy must be supported by the expertise of specialized personnel who are able to accurately monitor the course of the treatment itself.

8

APPETIZERS & SIDES

1) "Carrots" stuffed with cream cheese

INGREDIENTS:

- For the base:
- 1 1/2 cups almond flour
- 2 tablespoons psyllium husk
- 1/4 cup grated Parmesan cheese
- Salt and spices to taste
- 1 tablespoon apple cider vinegar
- 1/4 cup water
- 1 egg
- For the filling:
- 1 1/3 cups cream cheese
- Arugula for garnish

DIRECTIONS:

1. Beat the egg with the water and vinegar, add the Parmesan cheese, then the almond flour, salt and spices and finally the psyllium husk.
2. Knead and make a ball, then let stand in the fridge for 15 minutes. Divide the dough into 6 balls that you will roll out between 2 sheets of baking paper with the help of a rolling pin.
3. Fold the obtained disks to make carrot–shaped rolls and put them in cylindrical molds, previously buttered or lined with baking paper. Bake at 320° F (160° C) for 15 minutes.
4. Alternatively, this dough can also be fried. Stuff with cream cheese adding spices and salt and garnish with arugula leaves.

NUTRITION:

Calories 1138 Carbs 43g Fat 85g Protein 51g

2) Cauliflower and turmeric croquettes

INGREDIENTS:

- 1 cup boiled or steamed cauliflower
- 1 yolk
- 1 tablespoon bamboo flour
- Salt, pepper and turmeric
- 2 tablespoons grana cheese
- Parsley

DIRECTIONS:

1. Mash the cauliflower with a fork and, if it is still wet, squeeze it with your hands.
2. Add all the other ingredients and shape the croquettes.
3. Dip them in a beaten egg and then in bamboo flour.
4. Bake in the air fryer at 310° F (155° C) for 15 minutes or in the oven at 355° F (180° C) until golden brown.

NUTRITION:

Calories 137 Carbs 10g Fat 7g Protein 9g

3) Cauliflower popcorn

INGREDIENTS:

- ➢ 1 medium-sized cauliflower
- ➢ Paprika to taste
- ➢ Pink salt
- ➢ Pepper
- ➢ 1 1/2 tablespoons coconut oil or clarified butter

DIRECTIONS:

1. Wash and dry the cauliflower.
2. Break it into small pieces making sure to keep the florets intact.
3. Place them in a bowl, add the coconut oil, salt, pepper and paprika.
4. Mix and place in a baking sheet covered with baking paper.
5. Bake in the preheated fan oven at 355° F (180° C) for about 30/35 minutes.
6. Stir and bake for another 10 minutes in grill mode. Serve hot.

NUTRITION:

Calories 204 Carbs 5g Fat 20g Protein 2g

4) Cheese flans

INGREDIENTS:

- ➢ 1/2 cup Parmesan cheese
- ➢ 1/2 cup grated mozzarella cheese
- ➢ 1 egg

DIRECTIONS:

1. Mix all the ingredients together and pour the mixture into 6 molds.
2. Bake in the oven at 355° F (180° C) for 15 minutes.
3. Let cool and serve.

NUTRITION:

Calories 458 Carbs 4g Fat 33g Protein 36g

5) Chickpea breadsticks

INGREDIENTS for 20 breadsticks:

- ➢ 3/4 cup chickpea flour
- ➢ 2 1/2 cups water
- ➢ 1/2 cup coconut flour
- ➢ 1 tablespoon extra virgin olive oil
- ➢ Rosemary and thyme
- ➢ Pink salt

DIRECTIONS:

1. Bring the water to a boil with the salt and spices.
2. Add the flour and blend with the electric mixer to avoid lumps.
3. Cook for about 7 minutes until thickened. Place the dough on the baking paper and let cool.
4. Cut into 1/2 inch strips and bake in the oven at 390° F (200° C) for 20 minutes.

NUTRITION:

Calories 621 Carbs 72g Fat 27g Protein 9

6) Crispy baked chickpeas

INGREDIENTS for 2 people:

- ➢ 1 cup boiled chickpeas (or even canned chickpeas)
- ➢ 1 tablespoon extra virgin olive oil
- ➢ 1/2 teaspoon curry powder
- ➢ 1/2 teaspoon smoked paprika (or other spices if you do not like these)
- ➢ Salt and pepper to taste

DIRECTIONS:

1. Rinse the chickpeas several times and dry them.
2. Put them in a bowl and season them with curry and paprika, or with the spices you prefer.
3. Place the chickpeas in a nonstick baking sheet and distribute them well so that they do not overlap.
4. Bake them in the preheated oven at 390° F (200° C) in fan mode.
5. Let them toast for 1/2 hour, moving them from time to time. Let cool and enjoy.

NUTRITION:

Calories 417 Carbs 47g Fat 19g Protein 16

7) Crunchy mint-flavored zucchini chips

INGREDIENTS:

- ➤ 3 medium-sized zucchinis
- ➤ Extra virgin olive oil for frying
- ➤ Salt to taste
- ➤ Mint-flavored extra virgin olive oil

DIRECTIONS:

1. Wash and cut the zucchinis into thin rounds. Place some sheets of paper towel on the countertop, lay the zucchini rounds and pat dry.
2. Bring to the right temperature plenty of extra virgin olive oil for frying.
3. Cook the zucchini rounds in hot oil over medium heat taking care to turn them often until golden brown.
4. Once ready, place the crunchy fried zucchini chips on paper towel.
5. Let them cool slightly to acquire more crunchiness. Before serving, season with salt and a drizzle of mint-flavored oil.
6. It will give that intense, aromatic, fresh and pungent scent which is characteristic of fresh mint leaves.

NUTRITION:

Calories 228 Carbs 18g Fat 14g Protein 7g

8) Keto arancini (Sicilian specialty)

INGREDIENTS:

- ➤ For the dough:
- ➤ 14 ounces chicken
- ➤ 1/4 cup tomato sauce
- ➤ 2 tablespoons lupin flour
- ➤ 1 tablespoon almond flour
- ➤ Salt/pepper
- ➤ Oil
- ➤ For the filling:
- ➤ Smoked provola cheese
- ➤ Avocado

DIRECTIONS:

1. After chopping the chicken, add sauce, salt and black pepper and mix.
2. You can shape the arancini with your hands or with the appropriate tool.
3. Grease your hands or the tool with oil, take a bit of chicken, provola and avocado, then more chicken and shape small balls. Set aside and prepare the breadcrumbs by mixing flours with a little salt.
4. Brush the arancini with oil, bread them and put them on a baking sheet lined with baking paper. Brush them again with oil. Bake in the hot oven at 390° F (200° C) for 25/30 minutes.

NUTRITION:

Calories 660 Carbs 12g Fat 19g Protein 111g

9) Keto bagels

INGREDIENTS for 5 bagels:

- ➢ 1/2 cup golden flaxseed flour
- ➢ 1/4 cup almond flour
- ➢ 1 tablespoon Parmesan cheese
- ➢ 1 teaspoon yeast
- ➢ 1/2 cup egg whites
- ➢ 3 tablespoons extra virgin olive oil
- ➢ Salt, pepper and spices to taste (such as marjoram)
- ➢ Seeds for garnish

DIRECTIONS:

1. Mix the dry ingredients together. Separately, mix the liquid ingredients.
2. Combine the two mixtures. Fill the donut mold, but don't reach the edge.
3. Top with the seeds. Bake in microwave at 600 W for 3 minutes.
4. Then place the bagels on the microwave grill and grill for 7 minutes.
5. Let cool and stuff as you prefer, for example with cheese, ham, salad and a slice of tomato.

NUTRITION:

Calories 789 Carbs 8g Fat 66g Protein 42g

10) Keto canapé

INGREDIENTS:

- ➢ 2 raw fennels
- ➢ Slightly aged Pecorino cheese
- ➢ 10 slices salami

DIRECTIONS:

1. Wash the fennels and cut them into slices crosswise.
2. Use a ring mold to shape rounds of Pecorino cheese and put them on top of the fennel slices.
3. Add the salami slices and your delicious appetizer is ready!

NUTRITION:

Calories 314 Carbs 16g Fat 18g Protein 21g

11) Keto crackers

INGREDIENTS:

- ➢ 1 cup almond flour
- ➢ 3/4 cup grated Emmental cheese
- ➢ 1 egg
- ➢ Salt to taste
- ➢ Spices to taste (sesame, chives, paprika)

DIRECTIONS:

1. Mix all the dry ingredients and finally add the egg.
2. With the help of a rolling pin, roll out the dough obtained between two sheets of baking paper and add more spices on the surface if you like it.
3. Bake for 10/15 minutes at 340° F (170° C) in the preheated oven.
4. Let cool down and cut into small squares. Here are your keto crackers!
5. NUTRITION:
6. Calories 564 Carbs 3g Fat 44g Protein 39g

12) Keto finger foods (fried salmon and vegetables)

INGREDIENTS:

- ➢ ounces salmon fillet cut into pieces
- ➢ Vegetables of your choice
- ➢ For the batter:
- ➢ 1 tablespoon bamboo fiber
- ➢ 1 tablespoon Adamsbro Backprotein (whey) by Pinkfoodshop
- ➢ 1 teaspoon xanthan gum
- ➢ 1/2 teaspoon pink salt
- ➢ Warm water

DIRECTIONS:

1. Mix all the ingredients for the batter to obtain a thick mixture (it will make fish and vegetables as crispy as tempura!).
2. Shape carrot, celery and eggplant rounds.
3. Dip the salmon pieces and vegetable rounds in the batter.
4. Fry in very hot coconut oil. Enjoy with mayonnaise and mustard.

NUTRITION:

Calories 309 Carbs 5g Fat 15g Protein 40g

13) Keto frankfurter sausage rolls

INGREDIENTS for about 36 rolls:

- 3 cups KFT flour
- 1/4 cup bamboo fiber
- 2 eggs
- 1 sachet yeast
- 1/4 cup soft butter
- 2 tablespoons erythritol
- 3/4 cup milk
- 2 teaspoons salt

DIRECTIONS:

1. First dissolve the yeast with 1/4 cup of milk and 3/4 tablespoon of erythritol.
2. Mix the flours, add the dissolved yeast, the remaining erythritol and milk.
3. Mix in the kneader and add the eggs one at a time, then the salt and butter little by little.
4. Once the dough is smooth and soft, let it rise for about an hour.
5. Roll it out to obtain a thickness of half a cm, shape strips and wrap the pieces of sausage (if you buy the big ones, you can make 4 pieces out of one).
6. Let the rolls rise for another hour, brush with beaten egg and bake at 355° F (180° C) for about 20-30 minutes (until browned).

NUTRITION:

Calories 988 Carbs 96g Fat 56g Protein 26g

14) Keto fries (Apulian specialty)

INGREDIENTS:

- 1 cup almond flour
- 3/4 cup egg whites
- 2 tablespoons extra virgin olive oil
- 1 teaspoon yeast
- 1 teaspoon salt
- Oregano to taste

DIRECTIONS:

1. Blend the almond flour and oil in a food processor or with a hand whisk. Add yeast, salt and oregano using the mixer once more. Gradually add the egg whites while mixing the dough until it is well blended.
2. Don't overwork the dough. Don't worry: if it is lumpy and semi-liquid, that's how it should be. In the oven the "magic" will happen.
3. Use a donut mold if you want to make the classic frise with the hole in the middle.
4. Otherwise, you can use any muffin mold. Bake at 355° F (180° C) for 15 minutes, until golden brown. Let cool, cut the frise in half and bake in the oven (grill mode) for another 8/10 minutes.
5. When cold, dress the frise with cherry tomato and oregano salad and plenty of extra virgin olive oil.

NUTRITION:

Calories 460 Carbs 2g Fat 39g Protein 24g

15) Keto muffins with smoked salmon

INGREDIENTS for 4 muffins:

- 1/4 cup almond flour
- 1 tablespoon coconut flour
- 1/4 cup Parmesan cheese
- 1 teaspoon yeast
- Salt to taste
- 1 egg
- 1/4 cup linseed oil
- 1/4 cup white yogurt
- 1 1/2 tablespoons coconut milk
- 2 ounces smoked salmon

DIRECTIONS:

1. Preheat the oven to 355° F (180° C) in static mode. In a bowl, mix all dry ingredients. In another one, mix all liquid ingredients. Combine the two mixtures and stir until you get a homogeneous mixture.
2. Add the chopped salmon and mix again to distribute it throughout the mixture.
3. Brush the muffin molds with butter and fill them with the mixture.
4. Leave a few millimeters below the rim of the molds. Top with poppy seeds and a small piece of salmon. Bake for 20 minutes. Once baked, let them cool before removing them from the molds.
5. If you like, you can garnish them with a cream of cheese, extra virgin olive oil, salt and pepper.

NUTRITION:

Calories 285 Carbs 14g Fat 15g Protein 25g

16) Keto muffins with zucchini and bacon

INGREDIENTS:

- 1 whole egg + 1 egg white
- 1/2 cup almond flour
- 1/4 cup Backprotein flour by KetoChef
- 1 large zucchini
- 1/4 cup diced bacon
- 1 teaspoon olive oil
- Salt and spices to taste
- 1 teaspoon yeast
- Sparkling water if needed

DIRECTIONS:

1. First, clean the zucchini and cut it into small cubes, then add the diced bacon.
2. In a bowl, beat the whole egg and egg white, add a teaspoon of olive oil and season with salt and spices to taste. Stir in the almond flour, Backprotein flour and yeast. Incorporate the zucchini and bacon.
3. The mixture should be soft, so add a little sparkling water if necessary.
4. Place the mixture in baking cups or a muffin mold and bake in the fan oven for 20/30 minutes at 340° F (170° C).
5. Once baked, enjoy the softness and distinct flavor of these mouthwatering muffins.
6. N.B: If you don't have Backprotein flour, you can replace it with 1/4 cup of almond or coconut flour, obviously the result will change slightly.
7. Backprotein flours are suitable for sweet or savory dishes and can replace up to half of other types of flour, making the dough much fluffier and risen.

NUTRITION:

Calories 654 Carbs 17g Fat 43g Protein 49g

17) Keto pizza rolls

INGREDIENTS:

- ➢ For the dough:
- ➢ 2 cups RevoMix Pizza & Calzoni flour by Revolution03
- ➢ 3/4 cup cold water
- ➢ 1 1/2 tablespoons seed oil
- ➢ 1/2 teaspoon salt
- ➢ For the filling:
- ➢ ounces cooked ham
- ➢ 1 cup provola cheese

DIRECTIONS:

1. Knead the ingredients and let rise for 90 minutes.
2. Roll out the dough with the help of a rolling pin, shape a rectangle and stuff with ham and provola.
3. Roll up, cut into pieces of about 1.5/2 inches and place them in a baking sheet, well-spaced (you can also use the muffin pan).
4. Bake in the preheated static oven at 390° F (200° C) for 30 minutes.

NUTRITION:

Calories 844 Carbs 5g Fat 56g Protein 81g

18) Keto rustici (Apulian snack)

INGREDIENTS:

- ➢ 1 cup RevoMix Pasta flour by Revolution03
- ➢ 1/3 cup water
- ➢ 1 tablespoon soft butter
- ➢ 2 pinches salt
- ➢ 1 teaspoon brewer's yeast
- ➢ Egg yolk

DIRECTIONS:

1. Knead and roll out to obtain a thin sheet.
2. Make the shapes you like and let rustici rise for 1 hour or more.
3. Preheat the oven to 355° F (180° C) in static mode, brush the rustici with the egg yolk mixture and bake for 20 minutes.
4. Stuff as you like.

NUTRITION:

Calories 428 Carbs 7g Fat 17g Protein 63g

19) Keto taralli with fennel seeds (Apulian specialty)

INGREDIENTS:

- ➢ 1 cup almond flour
- ➢ 1/2 cup Parmesan cheese
- ➢ 1 tablespoon psyllium husk
- ➢ 1 egg
- ➢ 1 tablespoon extra virgin olive oil
- ➢ Salt to taste
- ➢ Fennel seeds to taste

DIRECTIONS:

1. Mix all the dry ingredients, then add the oil and egg.
2. Knead everything together with your hands. Once obtained a compact dough, let stand in the fridge for 5 minutes.
3. After that, shape your taralli on a sheet of baking paper by dividing the dough into small rolls and giving them the classic ring shape.
4. Bake in the preheated oven at 355° F (180° C) for 15 minutes until golden brown. Let cool down before serving.

NUTRITION:

Calories 566 Carbs 9g Fat 46g Protein 29g

20) Keto tortillas

INGREDIENTS:

- ➤ 1 cup almond flour
- ➤ 1/4 cup coconut flour
- ➤ 1 teaspoon psyllium
- ➤ 1 egg
- ➤ 1 tablespoon apple cider vinegar
- ➤ 1/2 teaspoon baking soda
- ➤ tablespoons water
- ➤ Dehydrated onion
- ➤ Salt

DIRECTIONS:

1. Mix all the dry ingredients together. Mix the egg and all the liquid ingredients.
2. Let stand for 10 minutes. Put the dough between 2 sheets of baking paper and roll out.
3. Cut into triangles and bake at 355° F (180° C) for 30 minutes. Be careful because the cooking time is closely related to the thickness of your tortillas: the thinner they are, the less they must remain in the oven.
4. Always check and let them cool in the oven before salting them.
5. You can enjoy them with arugula and avocado cream.

NUTRITION:

Calories 343 Carbs 23 Fat 21g Protein 16g

21) Low carb keto empanadas (Spanish/Latin-American pastry turnovers)

INGREDIENTS:

- ➤ For the dough:
- ➤ 2 cups RevoMix Pizza flour by Revolution03
- ➤ 1 cup boiling water
- ➤ 1/4 cup ghee
- ➤ 1 teaspoon salt
- ➤ For the filling:
- ➤ 1 cup coarse minced meat
- ➤ 2 1/2 cups spring onions
- ➤ 1 green bell pepper
- ➤ 2 hard-boiled eggs
- ➤ 10 olives
- ➤ Salt and pepper to taste
- ➤ Sweet paprika to taste
- ➤ Cumin to taste

DIRECTIONS:

1. Place all ingredients in the kneader and knead for about 3 minutes.
2. Let the dough stand for an hour in the fridge, then roll it out (you can use a dough sheeter or a rolling pin) to obtain a thickness of about half a cm.
3. Shape some discs to be filled.
4. Sauté spring onions and peppers with a little bit of extra virgin olive oil.
5. Add the meat and a tablespoon of ghee, salt, pepper, paprika and cumin. Add half a cup of water and simmer. Allow to cool and then add the hard-boiled eggs, olives and the remains of the spring onions (the green part).
6. Stir and the filling for the discs will be ready. Shape the pastry turnovers and bake in the oven at 430° F (220° C).

NUTRITION:

Calories 778 Carbs 12g Fat 45g Protein 81g

22) Low carb&fat pizza bites

INGREDIENTS:

- ➤ For the dough:
- ➤ 3/4 cup RevoMix flour by Revolution03
- ➤ 1/4 cup water
- ➤ 1 pinch salt
- ➤ For garnish:
- ➤ Skyrella cheese and tomato with spices

DIRECTIONS:

1. Mix all the ingredients and knead.
2. Let stand for an hour (if you have time, even more).
3. With a ring mold, shape small pizzas (about 10/12).
4. Bake in the fan oven at 355° F (180° C) for 15/20 minutes and garnish.

NUTRITION:

Calories 515 Carbs 26g Fat 15g Protein 71g

23) Parmesan "clouds"

INGREDIENTS for about 10 little clouds:

- Egg white of 1 medium-sized egg
- 2 cups grated Parmesan cheese
- Pepper to taste

DIRECTIONS:

1. Mix all the ingredients together and shape small balls (don't make them too big because then they grow).
2. Put in the fridge for 15 minutes.
3. Fry in the air fryer on baking paper at 355° F (180° C) for 12 minutes and after half the time turn them a little bit (check the cooking anyway).

NUTRITION:

Calories 896 Carbs 8g Fat 64g Protein 72g

24) Supplì (Italian rice balls with tomato sauce)

INGREDIENTS for 30 small or 15 large supplì:

- For the dough:
- 1 1/2 cups rice
- 1/3 cup butter
- 1/2 cup Grana Padano cheese
- 1 cup tomato puree
- Extra virgin olive oil
- 1 garlic clove
- Basil
- 1/2 cup smoked provola cheese
- Salt and pepper to taste
- For the breading:
- 3 eggs
- 2/3 cup low carb breadcrumbs
- Salt

DIRECTIONS:

1. Boil the rice and prepare a tomato and basil sauce (garlic is optional).
2. Melt the butter in the still hot rice, then add the other ingredients. Let the mixture cool in the fridge for at least 1 hour.
3. Shape the supplì, bread them and lay them on a baking sheet lined with baking paper.
4. Sprinkle with a little bit of extra virgin olive oil and bake in the hot oven at 390° F (200° C) for 15-20 minutes. Let cool.
5. You can freeze them, so that they will be ready to fry whenever you feel like it. If you want to eat them immediately, fry them directly, in extra virgin olive oil or in the air fryer.

NUTRITION:

Calories 1228 Carbs 77g Fat 83g Protein 44g

25) Tomini with bacon and walnuts

INGREDIENTS for 4 people:

- tomini (small Italian tomino cheese rounds)
- 1/4 cup diced smoked bacon
- 4 walnut kernels

DIRECTIONS:

1. Cut off the top of the tomini.
2. Put bacon and walnuts on them.
3. Bake at 320° F (160° C) for 12/15 minutes.

NUTRITION:

Calories 501 Carbs 2g Fat 41g Protein 30g

9

BREAKFAST RECIPES

1) Almond cake

INGREDIENTS:

- ➢ 1/4 cup oat flour
- ➢ 1/2 cup almond flour
- ➢ 1 tablespoon bamboo fiber
- ➢ 4 teaspoons erythritol
- ➢ 1 level teaspoon baking powder
- ➢ 3/4 cup egg whites
- ➢ 1 handful almonds
- ➢ Erythritol powder for garnish

DIRECTIONS:

1. Combine the dry ingredients, then add the egg whites slowly and mix with the help of a whisk. You will get a soft and sticky mixture.
2. Finally, add the whole almonds with skin.Pour into a small plum cake mold (for example a 3 x 7-in mold), put more almonds to decorate and bake at 355° F (180° C) for 30 minutes.
3. Test with the toothpick to make sure it is dry. Once cooled, sprinkle with erythritol powder.

NUTRITION:

Calories 538 Carbs 29g Fat 31g Protein 37g

2) Almond cookies with extra dark chocolate

INGREDIENTS for 24 cookies:

- ➢ 2 cups peeled almonds
- ➢ 1/4 cup butter
- ➢ 1/4 cup erythritol
- ➢ 1 egg
- ➢ 1 teaspoon cinnamon
- ➢ Extra dark chocolate 90% or more

DIRECTIONS:

1. Put the almonds, erythritol and cinnamon in a blender and blend until you get the consistency of flour.
2. Add the egg and butter in small pieces and blend again.
3. Shape 24 balls with the dough obtained and put them on a plate lined with baking paper. Crush the balls to give a round shape, put a small piece of extra dark chocolate on them and bake in the oven at 355° F (180° C) for 12-15 minutes. Let cool.

NUTRITION:

Calories 1688 Carbs 10g Fat 161g Protein 51g

3) Baked oats with pecan, raisin and cinnamon double layer

INGREDIENTS:

- For the base:
- 1/4 cup oats
- 1/3 cup Backprotein flour
- 1 cup plant milk
- 1 tablespoon raisins
- Pecans
- Egg
- Cinnamon
- For the filling:
- Yoeggs protein pudding
- 1 tablespoon pecans
- Pecans and cinnamon topping

DIRECTIONS:

1. Mix the oats, flour, milk, raisins and cinnamon together obtaining a thick mixture. Pour into two baking cups and bake for 15 minutes.
2. Remove from the baking cups, top with the pudding in which you have crumbled pecans and complete with the second layer, pecans and cinnamon.

NUTRITION:

Calories 787 Carbs 56g Fat 32g Protein 69g

4) Bamboo and avocado pancakes

INGREDIENTS:

- 2 eggs
- 1/2 ripe avocado
- 1 tablespoon bamboo fiber
- 1 tablespoon oat fiber
- 1 teaspoon xanthan
- 1/4 cup water
- 1/2 teaspoon instant yeast
- 1 pinch salt

DIRECTIONS:

1. Mash the avocado and blend it with the eggs.

2. Mix with water a little at a time.
3. Adjust the mixture to make it "doughy", not liquid. Add the dry ingredients avoiding lumps.
4. Grease a pancake pan and cook.

NUTRITION:

Calories 298 Carbs 4g Fat 24g Protein 15g

5) Blueberry and raspberry plum cake

INGREDIENTS:

- 1 3/4 cups almond flour
- 1/4 cup coconut flour
- 1 pinch salt
- 1 sachet (1/2 tablespoon) cream of tartar
- 1/2 cup fresh cream
- 2 eggs
- 1/4 cup erythritol
- Blueberries and raspberries to taste

DIRECTIONS:

1. Simply combine all ingredients.
2. Mix well and place in a plum cake mold. Put the fruit on the surface, so that some blueberries and raspberries go to the center of the cake.
3. Bake in the preheated oven at 355° F (180° C) for about 35 minutes.
4. Let cool before cutting.

NUTRITION:

Calories 1289 Carbs 60g Fat 91g Protein 59g

6) Braided pastries

INGREDIENTS for 4 braided pastries:

For the dough:

- 1/2 cup almond flour
- 1/2 cup bamboo fiber
- 1/3 cup erythritol
- 1 teaspoon vanilla
- 1 teaspoon xanthan
- 1 pinch salt
- 1/2 sachet baking powder
- 1/4 cup plant milk or sugar-free coconut milk (warm)
- 1/2 cup egg whites

For garnish:

- 1 tablespoon plant milk
- Powdered and granulated erythritol

DIRECTIONS:

1. Mix together all the dry ingredients, then add the egg whites.
2. Knead and pour the warm milk. Mix for a few minutes. Put the dough on the work surface, sprinkle with bamboo fiber and knead for a few more minutes.
3. Divide the dough into 4 parts, using each part to make an 8-10 inch long sausage.
4. Make a U and overlap the "legs" to form the braid.
5. Place the braids well-spaced on a baking sheet lined with baking paper. Bake in the preheated oven at 340° F (170° C) for 30 minutes.
6. Finally brush the braids with milk and plenty of granulated erythritol. Once cooled, you can add powdered erythritol.
7. For the chocolate version, simply roll the dough in dark chocolate sprinkles before making the braid.

NUTRITION:

Calories 384 Carbs 15g Fat 24g Protein 28g

7) Carrot and apple cookies

INGREDIENTS:

- 3/4 cup grated carrots
- 1/2 cup stevia
- tablespoons coconut oil
- 1/4 cup unsweetened apple compote
- 2 cups almond flour
- 1/4 cup psyllium flour
- Cardamom to taste
- 1 teaspoon baking powder
- 2 tablespoons dark chocolate chips
- 1 pinch salt
- Plant milk to taste

DIRECTIONS:

1. Mix the ingredients until you have a smooth and rich mixture.
2. Let stand in the fridge for 40 minutes. Then bake in the static oven at 355° F (180° C) for 25 minutes.
3. Check the cooking before taking out of the oven and enjoy.

NUTRITION:

Calories 1520 Carbs 108g Fat 99g Protein 50g

8) Cheese omelet

INGREDIENTS for one person:

- 2 eggs
- 1/4 cup cream
- salt and pepper
- 4 slices tomato
- 1/4 cup buffalo mozzarella
- Basil
- 1 tablespoon oil

DIRECTIONS:

1. Beat the eggs with the cream and season with salt and pepper.
2. Pour into hot oil and let it thicken slightly.
3. Place mozzarella, tomato and basil on top, let thicken and fold into an omelet.

NUTRITION:

Calories 407 Carbs 7g Fat 30g Protein 26g

9) Choco cereals

INGREDIENTS:

- ➤ 1 cup almond flour
- ➤ 1/4 cup erythritol
- ➤ 2 tablespoons bitter cocoa
- ➤ 1/4 cup butter
- ➤ Vanillin

DIRECTIONS:

1. Mix the dry ingredients and finally add the melted butter.
2. Shape a ball and place in the fridge covered with plastic wrap for 10 minutes.
3. Take the dough and shape small balls with your hands.
4. Place on a baking sheet covered with baking paper and bake in the preheated oven at 355° F (180° C) for 15 minutes.
5. Let cool before enjoying with almond milk or other plant milk of your choice.

NUTRITION:

Calories 1674 Carbs 42g Fat 149g Protein 41g

10) Choco-coffee stars

INGREDIENTS:

- ➤ 3/4 cup almond flour
- ➤ 1/2 cup chocolate 85%
- ➤ 2 tablespoons butter
- ➤ 2 tablespoons erythritol (such as Sauton)
- ➤ 1 espresso
- ➤ 1 tablespoon instant coffee
- ➤ 1/2 teaspoon baking powder
- ➤ 2 whole eggs

DIRECTIONS:

1. Whip the egg whites until stiff. With an electric mixer, blend the yolks with the erythritol.
2. Melt the chocolate and the espresso with the butter and add it to the yolks.
3. Dissolve the instant coffee in a little water and add it to the mixture.
4. Always with the help of the electric mixer, add the almond flour and egg whites.
5. Place in the baking cups and bake in the oven in a bain-marie for about 25/30 minutes.

NUTRITION:

Calories 1205 Carbs 39g Fat 99g Protein 40g

11) Chocolate pinwheels

INGREDIENTS:

- ➤ 1 cup RevoMix Pizza flour by Revolution03
- ➤ 3/4 tablespoon sunflower oil
- ➤ 1/4 cup powdered or liquid erythritol
- ➤ Warm water (to make a solid dough)
- ➤ Cocoa cream by Revolution03 for the filling

DIRECTIONS:

1. Make the dough and let it stand for 2 hours.
2. Roll out with a rolling pin to obtain a thin layer, cut into strips and let rise for another hour.
3. Stuff with the cream, roll up and bake at 355° F (180° C) for about 20 minutes.

NUTRITION:

Calories 192 Carbs 2g Fat 6g Protein 34g

12) Cocoa bombs

INGREDIENTS for 13 bombs of about 1/3 ounce:

- ➤ 1/3 cup cocoa
- ➤ 1/4 cup erythritol
- ➤ 1/4 cup Moka coffee
- ➤ 1/4 cup coconut oil
- ➤ 1/2 teaspoon cinnamon
- ➤ 1 pinch salt

DIRECTIONS:

1. Mix cocoa, erythritol, cinnamon and salt.
2. Add coffee and coconut oil and mix again. Shape small balls.
3. Enjoy or put in the fridge.

NUTRITION:

Calories 504 Carbs 6g Fat 53g Protein 2g

13) Coconut brownies

INGREDIENTS for one earthenware bowl:

For the base:

- ➢ 1/4 cup melted dark chocolate
- ➢ 2 eggs
- ➢ 1 teaspoon xylitol
- ➢ 1/4 cup degreased coconut flour
- ➢ 3/4 tablespoon coconut oil (in the chocolate)
- ➢ Coconut oil to taste (to grease the bowl)

For the topping:

- ➢ Coconut slices to taste
- ➢ 2 or 3 teaspoons coconut puree

DIRECTIONS:

1. Lightly beat the eggs and add the ingredients into the kneader one at a time.
2. Finish mixing with a spoon and the mixture will be very thick. Grease the bowl and put the mixture leveling it.
3. Garnish with the coconut slices and bake in the fan oven on the bottom rack at 320° F (160° C) for 20 minutes.
4. Let cool slightly and garnish with the soft coconut puree. You can eat it with coconut milk and water by Isola Bio.
5. Serve hot. If you can't, heat a piece in the microwave for 30 seconds.

NUTRITION:

Calories 481 Carbs 20g Fat 32g Protein 17g

14) Croissants

INGREDIENTS for 6 croissants:

- ➢ 1/2 cup almond flour
- ➢ 1/4 cup bamboo fiber
- ➢ 1 tablespoon coconut flour
- ➢ 1 tablespoon psyllium husk
- ➢ 1/4 cup erythritol
- ➢ 1/2 teaspoon vanilla
- ➢ 1/2 teaspoon xanthan
- ➢ 2 teaspoons bitter cocoa
- ➢ 1 pinch salt
- ➢ 1/2 tablespoon baking powder
- ➢ 1/2 cup egg whites
- ➢ 1/4 cup almond milk (lukewarm)
- ➢ To garnish:
- ➢ Jam
- ➢ Erythritol powder

DIRECTIONS:

1. Mix all the dry ingredients. Add the egg whites and begin to knead with your hands.
2. Pour in the milk and knead for a few more minutes. Let stand for 5 minutes.
3. Meanwhile, preheat the oven to 340° F (170° C).
4. With a rolling pin, roll out the dough between two sheets of baking paper to obtain a thickness of about 4 mm.
5. Cut out long triangles and roll them on themselves from the base, thus obtaining the shape of the croissant.
6. Place them on a baking sheet lined with baking paper, well-spaced. Bake for 15 minutes and garnish as you like.
7. You can cut them in half or use a pastry bag. Top them with some homemade jam (for example berry jam) and cream made with 1 tablespoon of mascarpone cheese, 1/2 tablespoon of sour cream (or yogurt), vanilla and erythritol to taste.

NUTRITION:

Calories 436 Carbs 23g Fat 27g Protein 30g

15) Egg in avocado

INGREDIENTS:

- 1 ripe avocado
- 2 eggs
- Salt and pepper

DIRECTIONS:

1. Cut the avocado in half and remove some of the flesh.
2. In a small bowl, gently open 1 egg at a time, then pour it into the avocado, being careful not to break the yolk (the egg may not fit all the way in).
3. Repeat the same steps for the other half; bake in the oven at 390° F (200° C) for 15 minutes. Season to taste with salt, pepper, chili pepper etc.

NUTRITION:

Calories 425 Carbs 3g Fat 39g Protein 17g

16) Espresso donuts

INGREDIENTS for 4 donuts:

- 1 cup almond flour
- 1 tablespoon amaretto-flavored espresso
- 1/2 tablespoon baking powder
- 1/3 cup powdered erythritol
- 1 egg
- 1/3 cup Greek yogurt
- 1 tablespoon lactose-free cream

DIRECTIONS:

1. Mix all the dry ingredients in a large bowl.
2. In another bowl, mix the egg with the yogurt and cream, removing all lumps.
3. Finally combine the two mixtures and bake in the fan oven at 340° F (170° C) for 25 minutes.

NUTRITION:

Calories 708 Carbs 20g Fat 49g Protein 37g

17) Flaxseed cookies

INGREDIENTS:

- 1/2 cup flaxseed flour
- 1/2 scoop collagen
- 1/2 scoop baking powder
- 3 tablespoons coconut oil
- 2 eggs
- Flavoring (such as Bulk)
- 1 pinch salt

DIRECTIONS:

1. Mix together all dry ingredients. Mix together all the liquids.
2. Then mix the two mixtures and shape the cookies. Bake at 355° F (180 ° C) for 10 minutes.

NUTRITION:

Calories 845 Carbs 23g Fat 70g Protein 31g

18) Flourless pancake tower

INGREDIENTS:

- 3 egg whites
- 2 yolks
- 1 tablespoon erythritol
- 1 scoop Chokkino cocoa
- Yumah cream for garnish

DIRECTIONS:

1. In a bowl, beat the egg yolks with erythritol and cocoa.
2. Gently add the egg whites previously beaten until stiff. Mix from the bottom up being careful not to disassemble the mixture.
3. With the help of a spoon, shape the pancakes in a hot nonstick pan (to make them perfect you can use silicone molds).
4. Garnish with Yumah cream and fresh raspberries.

NUTRITION:

Calories 185 Carbs 5g Fat 11g Protein 17g

19) Hazelnut, coconut and cocoa nib cookies

INGREDIENTS:

- ➤ 1 cup hazelnut flour
- ➤ 1/4 cup coconut flour
- ➤ 1/4 cup melted butter
- ➤ 1/4 cup egg whites
- ➤ 1 tablespoon erythritol
- ➤ 1 pinch salt
- ➤ 1 tablespoon cocoa nibs or chopped dark chocolate

DIRECTIONS:

1. Mix all the ingredients together and shape small balls.
2. Press them a little bit, bake in the hot oven at 355° F (180° C) for 15 minutes.
3. Garnish them with melted dark chocolate and a small piece of butter (optional).

NUTRITION:

Calories 699 Carbs 32g Fat 56g Protein 17g

20) Hazelnut donuts

INGREDIENTS for 2 donuts:

- ➤ 1/2 cup toasted hazelnut flour
- ➤ 1/4 cup erythritol (or less)
- ➤ 1 egg

DIRECTIONS:

1. Separate the yolk from the egg white.
2. Beat the yolk with the sugar in a bowl and the egg white in another one until stiff.
3. Add the flour to the whipped yolk and finally add the egg white.
4. Bake for 20 minutes at 320° F (160° C).

NUTRITION:

Calories 256 Carbs 4g Fat 23g Protein 8g

21) Hug cookies

INGREDIENTS:

- ➤ 1 cup almond flour
- ➤ 1 egg
- ➤ 1/4 cup erythritol
- ➤ 1/4 cup fresh cream
- ➤ 1 tablespoon ghee
- ➤ 1/3 cup bitter cocoa powder

DIRECTIONS:

1. Place all the ingredients in a bowl except cocoa.
2. Knead until the mixture is smooth. Divide it in half. In one half, add the cocoa powder.
3. Put in the baking cups half of one mixture and half of the other.
4. Bake at 355° F (180° C) for 25 minutes.

NUTRITION:

Calories 1030 Carbs 28g Fat 88g Protein 32g

22) Keto brownies with walnuts and orange peel

INGREDIENTS:

➢ 5 large eggs at room temperature
➢ 1/4 cup melted and cooled butter
➢ 1/4 cup Live Better coconut flour
➢ 1/4 cup almond or hazelnut flour
➢ 1/4 cup Live Better cocoa
➢ 1/2 teaspoon baking powder
➢ 1/4 cup Live Better fine erythritol
➢ 1/2 cup walnuts or pecans, coarsely chopped
➢ Orange peel (optional)

DIRECTIONS:

1. Preheat the oven to 355° F (180° C).
2. Mix the eggs and the now cold butter (otherwise it will cook the eggs) in a bowl or in the kneader.
3. Prepare the dry ingredients in another bowl: sift together the coconut flour, almond flour, baking powder, cocoa and erythritol and mix with a spoon.
4. Mix the dry ingredients, a little at a time, with the egg and butter mixture and mix until you get a smooth dough.
5. Add the coarsely chopped walnuts and orange peel and mix.
6. Line a baking sheet with baking paper. Pour in the dough in the shape of a square or rectangle, level with the spoon to obtain a thickness of about half an inch.
7. Bake for about 20 minutes, the surface should look firm and well cooked.
8. Do not overcook or the brownies will lose their internal softness. Let cool for 10 minutes, then cut into squares and put in the fridge for about 1 hour.

NUTRITION:

Calories 818 Carbs 20g Fat 66g Protein 37g

23) Keto cantucci (Tuscan almond cookies)

INGREDIENTS:

➢ 1 cup almond flour
➢ 1/2 cup pistachios, almonds, cranberries
➢ 1/4 cup erythritol
➢ 1 teaspoon baking powder
➢ 1 medium-sized egg
➢ Almond extract

DIRECTIONS:

1. Mix the solid ingredients, add the egg and almond extract.
2. Knead the dough and shape a 10-inch-long sausage.
3. Bake in the hot oven at 345° F (175° C) for 25 minutes.
4. Let cool completely and cut diagonally to shape the cookies (half a cm).
5. Put again in the oven at 345° F (175° C) for another 10/12 minutes. Enjoy by dipping them in cappuccino.

NUTRITION:

Calories 658 Carbs 24g Fat 49g Protein 30g

24) Keto churros (Spanish fried pastries)

INGREDIENTS:

- ➤ 2/3 cup almond flour
- ➤ 1/4 cup coconut flour
- ➤ 1 tablespoon psyllium flour
- ➤ 1 teaspoon xanthan
- ➤ 1 cup water
- ➤ 1/4 cup butter
- ➤ 2 tablespoons erythritol or 6 drops sweetener
- ➤ 1 pinch salt
- ➤ 2 beaten eggs
- ➤ Erythritol and cinnamon

DIRECTIONS:

1. Mix the flours and xanthan in a bowl. In a small pan, heat the water, butter, erythritol and salt
2. . When it's about to boil, add the flours in two batches and cook, stirring for a few minutes.
3. It should become a ball that pulls away from the edges.
4. Let cool a bit and add the eggs one at a time (do not add the second one if the first one has not been completely absorbed).
5. Pour the dough into a sac a poche with a star nozzle and on a baking sheet make 2-3 inch strips.
6. At this point you can fry them like classic churros or bake them in the hot oven at 355° F (180° C) for 10/12 minutes.

NUTRITION:

Calories 574 Carbs 30g Fat 36g Protein 29g

25) Keto granola

INGREDIENTS:

- ➤ 1/2 cup almonds
- ➤ 1/3 cup pumpkin seeds
- ➤ 1/4 cup sunflower seeds
- ➤ 1/3 cup shredded coconut
- ➤ 1/3 cup walnuts
- ➤ 2 tablespoons erythritol
- ➤ 1 teaspoon salt
- ➤ 1 teaspoon cinnamon
- ➤ 1 teaspoon vanillin

- ➤ 1/4 cup dark chocolate chips
- ➤ 1 egg white
- ➤ 2 tablespoons clarified butter

DIRECTIONS:

1. Place almonds, walnuts, seeds, chocolate and coconut in a blender and crumble a bit.
2. Add erythritol, salt, vanillin and cinnamon, then pour butter and egg whites.
3. Mix, pour the mixture on the baking paper and distribute all over the baking sheet to obtain a thickness of 5-7 mm.
4. Bake at 345° F (175° C) for about 15 minutes (until golden brown). Let cool and break into small pieces. Store the granola in a glass container.
5. You can increase or decrease the dry ingredients as you like.

NUTRITION:

Calories 744 Carbs 16g Fat 64g Protein 26g

26) Keto lebkuchen (German Christmas cookies)

INGREDIENTS for 6 lebkuchen:

- ➤ 1 cup almond flour
- ➤ 1/3 cup whole almond flour
- ➤ 1 tablespoon bamboo fiber
- ➤ 1 teaspoon psyllium flour
- ➤ 2 tablespoons soft butter
- ➤ 1 egg
- ➤ 1/3 cup erythritol
- ➤ 1 sachet keto dark chocolate chips

DIRECTIONS:

1. In a bowl, mix all the flours and spices (if you can't find a ready-made mix, you can easily make it yourself).
2. Separately, mix the butter with the erythritol, add the egg always kneading and then the flours a little at a time.
3. Make a ball and let stand in the fridge.
4. Form the typical star, pretzel and heart shapes or what you like best, and bake at 355° F (180° C) for 15 minutes.
5. Melt the chocolate and frost your cookies.

NUTRITION:

Calories 690 Carbs 30g Fat 49g Protein 31g

27) Keto Nutella

INGREDIENTS:

- 1 cup toasted hazelnuts
- 1 tablespoon cocoa
- 2 tablespoons coconut oil
- 1 tablespoons erythritol (or to taste)

DIRECTIONS:

1. Very patiently blend the hazelnuts until they become a liquid cream.
2. Add the other ingredients in order of how they are listed.
3. Store in a jar. Once cooled, the cream will become thick.

NUTRITION:

Calories 437 Carbs 5g Fat 45g Protein 4g

28) Keto tartlets

INGREDIENTS for 4 tartlets:

For the base:

- 1/4 cup egg whites
- 1 1/2 tablespoons melted clarified butter
- 1/2 cup almond flour
- 1/4 cup hazelnut flour
- (Sweetener to taste, such as 4 drops hazelnut flavoring)

For the filling:

- 2 tablespoons Fage Greek yogurt 5%
- 1 tablespoon melted dark chocolate 99% (or protein hazelnut cream)

DIRECTIONS:

1. Mix the flours with the egg whites, melted butter, flavoring or sweetener.
2. The dough should be very moldable. Roll out into tartlet molds and bake at 355° F (180° C) for 15 minutes.
3. Mix the yogurt with the melted dark chocolate and stuff the tartlets when they have chilled. You can also use a bit of protein hazelnut cream.

NUTRITION:

Calories 842 Carbs 26g Fat 68g Protein 32g

29) Lemon porridge with nuts and blueberries

INGREDIENTS:

- 1/4 cup oat flour
- 1/3 cup sugar-free almond milk
- 1/4 cup water
- 5 drops Tic sweetener
- Lemon peel and a few drops lemon juice

DIRECTIONS:

1. Put everything in a small pan, stir trying to eliminate lumps, then simmer until it reaches the desired density.
2. Garnish as you prefer (for example with chopped hazelnuts and pistachios, almond slivers and coconut) and enjoy.

NUTRITION:

Calories 85 Carbs 15g Fat 2g Protein 3g

30) Low carb banana bread with chocolate chips

INGREDIENTS:

- 4 large eggs
- 2 small/medium-sized bananas
- 1/3 cup sugar-free almond milk or coconut milk
- 1/4 cup extra virgin olive oil
- 3/4 cup coconut flour
- 1 tablespoon stevia/erythritol
- 1 teaspoon instant yeast
- 1/2 cup sugar-free dark chocolate chips
- 1 teaspoon vanilla extract and cinnamon (optional)

DIRECTIONS:

1. Preheat the oven to 340° F (170° C). Mix the dry ingredients.
2. In a large bowl, beat the eggs, then add the mashed bananas and all the liquid ingredients. Mix until smooth.
3. Add the dry ingredients to the liquid ones. Pour the mixture in a plum cake mold lined with baking paper.
4. Bake for 45-50 minutes. Let cool for at least 15 minutes before removing from the mold.

NUTRITION:

Calories 684 Carbs 74g Fat 29g Protein 32g

31) Low carb pangoccioli (Italian soft rolls with chocolate chips)

INGREDIENTS for 3 pangoccioli:

- ➤ 1 cup RevoMix Pizza flour by Revolution03
- ➤ 1/3 cup water
- ➤ 1 tablespoon organic extra virgin olive oil
- ➤ 1/4 cup extra dark chocolate 85%, cut into small pieces
- ➤ 2 tablespoons erythritol
- ➤ 1 pinch vanillin

DIRECTIONS:

1. In a bowl, combine the flour, vanillin and erythritol with the water.
2. Blend with the electric mixer and slowly add the oil.
3. Once the dough is ready, knead it for a few moments with your hands until smooth and homogeneous and let stand for 1 hour.
4. Then add the chocolate, knead again and let stand for another hour. Divide the dough into 3 balls and bake at 355° F (180° C) for 15 minutes.

NUTRITION:

Calories 305 Carbs 19g Fat 12g Protein 31g

32) Low carb pistachio blondies

INGREDIENTS:

- ➤ For the base:
- ➤ 1/4 cup coconut flour
- ➤ 2 1/2 tablespoons oat flour
- ➤ 1 tablespoon defatted almond flour
- ➤ 1/2 cup egg whites
- ➤ 1/2 cup sugar-free almond milk
- ➤ 2 tablespoons lactose-free, low-fat quark cheese
- ➤ 1/2 teaspoon baking powder
- ➤ 1 teaspoon chopped pistachios
- ➤ For garnish:
- ➤ 1 tablespoon pistachio protein cream
- ➤ Fresh fruit to taste

DIRECTIONS:

1. Mix all the ingredients for the base in a bowl until smooth.
2. Pour into a rectangular container greased with coconut oil and sprinkle with the granola.
3. Bake at 355° F (180° C) for 15/20 minutes. Garnish with pistachio protein cream and fresh fruit.

NUTRITION:

Calories 303 Carbs 28g Fat 9g Protein 26g

33) Mug cake with cocoa beans and extra dark chocolate

INGREDIENTS:

- ➤ 1 tablespoon yellow butter
- ➤ 1 tablespoon coconut flour
- ➤ 1 egg
- ➤ 1 tablespoon erythritol
- ➤ 1/4 teaspoon baking powder
- ➤ Cocoa beans
- ➤ Extra dark chocolate

DIRECTIONS:

1. Melt the butter in a ceramic mug in the microwave.
2. Mix all the dry ingredients in a small bowl, then add the melted butter and finally the egg.
3. Mix everything together with a fork. Use the remaining butter in the bowl to butter it well on all sides, then pour in the dough.
4. Top with cocoa beans and extra dark chocolate.
5. Bake in the microwave for about 60-90 seconds or in the static oven at 355° F (180° C) for 12-15 minutes.

NUTRITION:

Calories 166 Carbs 8g Fat 11g Protein 8g

34) Multilayer glass

INGREDIENTS:

For the base:

- ➢ 1 teaspoon chia seeds
- ➢ 1 teaspoon collagen
- ➢ 1 teaspoon MCT oil
- ➢ 1 teaspoon coconut flour
- ➢ 1 teaspoon shredded coconut
- ➢ Warm water

For the cream:

- ➢ 1/2 cup Greek yogurt 5%
- ➢ 1 teaspoon coconut oil
- ➢ Melted chocolate 99% and a few chocolate drops
- ➢ Inca'Cao macadamia nut butter (Belgian quality) by Pinkfoodshop
- ➢ 5 almonds

DIRECTIONS:

1. Make a small dough with the ingredients for the base and place in a glass.
2. On the cold base, put a layer of yogurt (mixed with coconut oil), followed by the warm melted chocolate with the chocolate drops in between to make it crunchy, a new layer of yogurt and almonds and finally a generous teaspoon of macadamia nut butter.
3. Let it stand in the fridge overnight.

NUTRITION:

Calories 497 Carbs 17g Fat 39g Protein 20g

35) Orange and blueberry pancake

INGREDIENTS:

- ➢ 1/4 cup egg whites
- ➢ 1/3 cup almond flour
- ➢ 1 tablespoon orange peel powder
- ➢ 1 tablespoon erythritol (optional)
- ➢ 1/2 teaspoon baking powder
- ➢ 1/4 cup fresh blueberries

DIRECTIONS:

1. First mix all the dry ingredients.
2. Whip the egg whites until stiff and gently

add the dry ingredients.

3. Heat a nonstick pan and grease it with very little oil. Pour the mixture and cook for 1 minute per side.

NUTRITION:

Calories 205 Carbs 13g Fat 11g Protein 13g

36) Peanut butter cookies

INGREDIENTS:

- ➢ 1/4 cup peanut butter
- ➢ 1 egg
- ➢ 1 tablespoon oat fiber
- ➢ 99% extra dark chocolate to taste

DIRECTIONS:

1. Mix the first 3 ingredients, shape small balls and crush them to create the cookies.
2. Bake in the fan oven for 10 minutes at 340° F (170° C).
3. Allow to cool. Melt the chocolate and dip half of the cookie. (If you like, you can modify the recipe by adding sweetener).

NUTRITION:

Calories 278 Carbs 9g Fat 21g Protein 13g

37) Pistachio cookies with collagen

INGREDIENTS:

- 2/3 cup pistachio butter
- 1/3 cup almond flour
- 1 scoop collagen
- 1 egg
- 1 pinch salt
- Dark chocolate chips

DIRECTIONS:

1. Mix everything together.
2. Place the dough balls on a baking sheet lined with baking paper.
3. Press with a fork and top with chocolate chips. Bake at 355° F (180° C) for 12 minutes.

NUTRITION:

Calories 411 Carbs 15g Fat 28g Protein 25g

38) Pistachio French toast

INGREDIENTS:

- 2 slices fresh rye bread
- 1/4 cup Greek yogurt
- 3/4 tablespoon protein cream by Revolution03
- 1 tablespoon egg white and 1 tablespoon milk (or just egg white)
- Erythritol or sweetener (optional)
- Fruit to taste

DIRECTIONS:

1. Mix the egg white and milk with erythritol.
2. Soak the bread and cook it in a saucepan for a few minutes per side.
3. Fill with yogurt and cream and if you want fruit (for example banana).
4. Cover with more yogurt, cream and fruit and enjoy hot or cold.

NUTRITION:

Calories 209 Carbs 23g Fat 7g Protein 13g

39) Protein waffles

INGREDIENTS:

- 1/4 cup protein powder
- 1 egg + 1 egg white
- 1 tablespoon bamboo fiber
- 1 tablespoon erythritol
- Sugar-free almond milk to taste

DIRECTIONS:

1. Mix the ingredients together and transfer the mixture into a silicone waffle mold.
2. Bake in the fan oven at 320° F (160° C) for 20 minutes.

NUTRITION:

Calories 191 Carbs 4g Fat 5g Protein 32g

40) Red fruit bars

INGREDIENTS:

- 1/4 cup almonds
- 1/4 cup walnuts
- 1/4 cup hazelnuts
- 1/4 cup pumpkin seeds
- 1/2 cup shredded coconut
- 2 tablespoons erythritol
- 1/4 cup clarified butter
- 1 egg
- Vanilla flavoring
- Dried strawberries and blueberries to taste

DIRECTIONS:

1. Put the nuts, coconut and seeds in a blender and crumble a bit.
2. Add the erythritol and vanilla flavoring, then pour in the melted butter and egg. Mix and add the dried fruit.
3. Pour the mixture on the baking paper and spread all over the baking sheet to obtain a thickness of about 5-7 mm.
4. Cut into squares and fix the edges. Bake at 345° F (175° C) for about 15 minutes (until golden brown). Let cool.

NUTRITION:

Calories 946 Carbs 17g Fat 84g Protein 30g

41) Red fruit "clouds"

INGREDIENTS:

- 1 tablespoon vanilla-flavored protein
- 1/4 cup almond flour
- 1/2 teaspoon xanthan
- 1/2 teaspoon baking powder
- Sweetener to taste (for example 20 drops Tic)
- 1/4 cup egg whites
- Strawberries and blueberries

DIRECTIONS:

1. Mix the dry ingredients together and add the egg whites.
2. You will get a rather sticky dough. With the help of two spoons, shape some nests and place in the hollow the strawberries and blueberries.
3. Bake at 355° F (180° C) for about 15 minutes or until golden brown. Check the cooking. Serve hot or warm.

NUTRITION:

Calories 289 Carbs 12g Fat 12g Protein 35g

42) Rusks with hazelnut yogurt

INGREDIENTS:

1. 2 tablespoons Fage yogurt 5%
2. 2 teaspoons hazelnut cream 100%
3. 2 light rusks
4. 1 long espresso
5. Hazelnut and cocoa cream by Pinkfoodshop
6. Homemade granola

DIRECTIONS:

1. Mix the yogurt with the hazelnut cream and place in freezer for 20 minutes.
2. Wet the rusks with the espresso and then layer the yogurt and hazelnut cream.
3. Garnish as you like (for example with hazelnut and chocolate cream and granola).

NUTRITION:

Calories 244 Carbs 32g Fat 10g Protein 6g

43) Shortcrust pastry cookies

INGREDIENTS:

- 1/4 cup coconut flour
- 1/4 cup almond flour
- 1/4 cup melted butter
- 1/4 cup erythritol
- 2 egg whites
- The grated peel of 1 organic lemon
- 1 pinch salt

DIRECTIONS:

1. First mix the dry ingredients and then the liquid ones until you get a firm dough like shortcrust pastry.
2. Bake at 355° F (180° C) for 20 minutes.
3. You can top the cookies with some raspberry compote (to make it, cook raspberries, juice of 1 lemon, erythritol and agar over low heat for 5 minutes).

NUTRITION:

Calories 457 Carbs 22g Fat 33g Protein 17g

44) Slice of choco-granola cake

INGREDIENTS:

- 1/4 cup Kellogg's granola with no added sugar
- 1/3 cup RevoMix Cake flour by Revolution03
- 1/2 cup egg whites
- 1/2 cup Sojasun coconut yogurt
- Chocolate chips to taste
- Nellina Zero hazelnut cream by Revolution03 for the topping

DIRECTIONS:

1. Mix the flour and egg whites and cook in a small pan as if making a pancake.
2. Once cooked, cut into three pieces to form the various layers. Layer with yogurt and chocolate chips.
3. Finish with a yogurt topping covered with granola and hazelnut cream.

NUTRITION:

Calories 283 Carbs 32g Fat 9g Protein 18g

45) Walnut cookies

INGREDIENTS:

- ➢ 1 cup RevoMix Cake flour by Revolution03
- ➢ 1/3 cup soft butter (room temperature)
- ➢ 1 tablespoon powdered erythritol (such as Sukrin icing by Pinkfoodshop)
- ➢ 1 egg
- ➢ 1 sachet vanillin
- ➢ 1 handful coarsely chopped walnuts

DIRECTIONS:

1. Whip the butter with 1/2 tablespoon of erythritol for two minutes, add the egg and continue to whip for another minute.
2. Add the RevoMix Cake flour and vanillin, mix for 3 minutes.
3. Add the chopped walnuts and mix everything together.
4. The dough will be a bit sticky. With the help of a teaspoon, take a little bit of dough and shape small balls, then press them with the help of a fork.
5. Bake at 390° F (200° C) for about 18 minutes. Check the browning. Let cool completely and then sprinkle with a little powdered erythritol

NUTRITION:

Calories 349 Carbs 9g Fat 25g Protein 22g

10
DESSERTS

1) Apple pie

INGREDIENTS:

- ➢ 3 small organic apples
- ➢ 3 tablespoons chufa flour
- ➢ 4 tablespoons coconut flour
- ➢ 1/2 cup coconut oil
- ➢ 1/4 cup erythritol
- ➢ 3 egg whites
- ➢ 1 sachet baking powder
- ➢ Vanilla flavoring
- ➢ 1 pinch salt

DIRECTIONS:

1. Dice the apples keeping the peel. Blend them with coconut oil and vanilla until you obtain a puree.
2. In a bowl, beat the egg whites and erythritol with an electric mixer until frothy. Add the flours and the apple puree.
3. The mixture should be dense and without the water that apples often release (this also depends on the type of apples).
4. In this case, add more coconut flour but very gradually, so as not to make it too dry.
5. Bake at 355° F (180° C) for 40 minutes. Always do the toothpick test!

NUTRITION:

Calories 788 Carbs 50g Fat 59g Protein 15g

2) Avocado ice cream

INGREDIENTS:

- ➢ 2 avocados
- ➢ Juice of 1/2 lemon
- ➢ 1 cup liquid sugar-free fresh cream
- ➢ 1/2 cup erythritol or liquid sweetener
- ➢ 1/2 cup Greek yogurt 10% fat

DIRECTIONS:

1. Split the avocado in half and remove the stone and peel.
2. Put the avocado pulp in a blender, add the lemon juice and blend (you can also use an immersion blender).
3. Add the erythritol or liquid sweetener, fresh cream and Greek yogurt and continue blending until creamy.
4. Pour the mixture into ice cream molds and place in the freezer for 2-3 hours.
5. After that, you can serve your avocado ice cream or leave it in the freezer and enjoy later!

NUTRITION:

Calories 1410 Carbs 15g Fat 141g Protein 21g

3) Avocado mousse with two chocolates

INGREDIENTS for 3 servings:

- ➤ 1 ripe avocado
- ➤ 3/4 cup sugar-free coconut milk
- ➤ 4 scoops Live Better magic powder
- ➤ 2 scoops Live Better cocoa powder
- ➤ 4 scoops erythritol
- ➤ 1/4 cup sugar-free dark chocolate

DIRECTIONS:

1. Put all the ingredients together and blend with an immersion blender until very creamy.
2. You can either eat it right away or let stand in the fridge for a bit.

NUTRITION:

Calories 603 Carbs 35g Fat 48g Protein 8g

4) Aztec cake

INGREDIENTS:

- ➤ erythritol + sucralose (or Tic sweetener) to taste
- ➤ 1/4 cup chocolate 100%
- ➤ 1/2 cup bitter cocoa powder
- ➤ 1/4 cup clarified butter
- ➤ 3/4 cup chopped almonds
- ➤ 2 eggs
- ➤ 1 teaspoon chili pepper
- ➤ 2 teaspoons rum

DIRECTIONS:

1. Separate yolks and egg whites, whip the latter and mix the former with erythritol, sweetener and rum.
2. Then incorporate into the whipped egg whites.
3. Melt chocolate and butter in a bain-marie (or in the microwave) and add to the mixture.
4. Finally add the chopped almonds and cocoa powder using a spatula and a level teaspoon of chili pepper. Add sweetener to taste.
5. Transfer to a medium-sized mold (it should not be too shallow, a 6-inch mold should be fine) and bake at 300° F (150° C) for 30 minutes.

NUTRITION:

Calories 1234 Carbs 38g Fat 104g Protein 38g

5) Bicolor crumble pie with goat's milk cheese cream and blueberry jam

INGREDIENTS for 8 servings:

- ➤ For the white base:
- ➤ 1 cup lupin flour
- ➤ 1/2 cup erythritol
- ➤ 1/4 cup clarified butter
- ➤ 1 large egg
- ➤ For the dark base:
- ➤ 1 cup lupin flour
- ➤ 1/2 cup erythritol
- ➤ 2 1/2 tablespoons clarified butter
- ➤ 1/4 cup dark chocolate 90%, melted
- ➤ 1 large egg
- ➤ For the goat's milk cheese cream:
- ➤ 1/2 cup goat's milk cheese
- ➤ 1 tablespoon erythritol
- ➤ 1 egg
- ➤ 1/2 cup blueberry jam 100%

DIRECTIONS:

1. Mix all the ingredients for the white base, shape a ball and let stand in the fridge for about 30 minutes, covered with plastic wrap.
2. Mix all the ingredients for the dark base, shape a ball and let stand in the fridge for 30 minutes, covered with plastic wrap.
3. Roll out the dough with the help of a rolling pin and baking paper.
4. Press with your fingers, shape, decorate, in short do as you like. Mix the ingredients for the goat's milk cheese cream and spread on top of the dough.
5. Add some tablespoons of jam. Spread part of the dark base and bake at 355° F (180° C) for 20/25 minutes.

NUTRITION:

Calories 1259 Carbs 32g Fat 106g Protein 44g

6) Caramelized almonds

INGREDIENTS:

- 1 1/2 cups almonds
- 5 tablespoons erythritol
- A little sucralose, stevia or Tic sweetener
- (Cinnamon if you like it)

DIRECTIONS:

1. Put in a nonstick pan the almonds, sugar and a little sweetener to make it sweeter.
2. Let the sugar melt and then turn off the stove.
3. Stir until the sugar crystallizes again: some of it will stick to the almond and some of it won't.
4. Do this at least 3 times: all the sugar will gradually stick to the almond and darken a bit. Then let cool.

NUTRITION:

Calories 1074 Carbs 30g Fat 90g Protein 36g

7) Chiffon cake with fresh cheese cream and raspberry and basil coulis

INGREDIENTS for 4 cups:

For the base:

- 1 1/2 tablespoons ghee
- 3 tablespoons almond flour
- 1/2 teaspoon baking powder
- 2 eggs
- 2 teaspoons keto jam
- 1 teaspoon erythritol

For the coulis:

- 2 cups raspberries (macerated with lime, 2 tablespoons of erythritol and 2 of water)
- A few basil leaves
- 2 tablespoons water
- For the cheese cream:
- 1 cup quark cheese 40%
- 3/4 cup fresh cream
- Vanilla beans
- 2 tablespoons powdered erythritol

DIRECTIONS:

1. Mix all the ingredients for the base in a wide mug and cook in several rounds for 2 and a half minutes, without ever opening the pan.
2. Make the raspberry coulis by putting the raspberries in a small pan with a few basil leaves and 2 tablespoons of water.
3. Cook for a few minutes until the raspberries are flavored with the basil. Remove the leaves and let cool.
4. For the cheese cream, whip together the cream with the quark cheese, erythritol and vanilla beans.
5. Compose the cup by putting in layers a slice of chiffon cake, some raspberry coulis and cheese cream. Complete with chopped chocolate and raspberry powder.

NUTRITION:

Calories 669 Carbs 41g Fat 46g Protein 22g

8) Chocolate pudding with full-fat thick coconut milk and hazelnuts

INGREDIENTS:

- 1 cup coconut milk
- 3 generous tablespoons organic, fair-trade, bitter cocoa powder
- 2 level teaspoons erythritol (zero glycemic index! Adjust according to your tolerance to sweet flavors)
- 1 teaspoon 100% organic, natural hazelnut paste (the label should indicate only hazelnuts, possibly salt and hazelnut oil, not sweetened hazelnuts or worse the various Nutellas!)
- 1 tablespoon chopped hazelnuts
- 1 teaspoon agar-agar powder

DIRECTIONS:

1. Dissolve the agar-agar powder in 1/2 inch of semi-boiling water at 175/195° F (80/90° C).
2. Mix all the ingredients except the chopped hazelnuts.
3. Place in a small bowl and let stand in the fridge for at least 2 hours.
4. Serve with the chopped hazelnuts or coconut flakes.

NUTRITION:

Calories 162 Carbs 14g Fat 10g Protein 4g

9) Chocolate "rafts"

INGREDIENTS:

- ➢ 2 cups almond flour
- ➢ 3/4 cup hazelnut flour
- ➢ 1 whole egg
- ➢ 1/4 cup erythritol
- ➢ 1 1/2 tablespoons orange peel powder
- ➢ 1/4 cup melted butter

DIRECTIONS:

1. Mix all the dry ingredients together, then mix the liquids.
2. Let the mixture stand in the fridge for 10 minutes. Roll out between 2 sheets of baking paper.
3. Cut out discs and shape them into small rafts by folding them with your fingers. Bake at 345° F (175° C) for 15 minutes.
4. Once cooled, stuff them as you like (for example with melted chocolate 85%, some compote or keto custard).

NUTRITION:

Calories 1663 Carbs 50g Fat 138g Protein 55g

10) Chocolate roll with blueberries

INGREDIENTS:

For the base:

- ➢ 1/2 cup egg whites
- ➢ 1/4 cup bitter cocoa powder
- ➢ 3 drops Tic or another sweetener to taste

For the filling:

- ➢ 1/4 cup Greek yogurt
- ➢ 10 blueberries

DIRECTIONS:

1. Blend the egg whites with the cocoa and sweetener and pour the mixture into a nonstick pan, greased with coconut oil.
2. Cook the crêpe and fill with yogurt and blueberries.
3. Roll it up and let it stand in the fridge overnight.

NUTRITION:

Calories 194 Carbs 19g Fat 3g Protein 23g

11) Chufa and blueberry pastries

INGREDIENTS:

- ➢ 1 cup chufa flour
- ➢ 1/4 cup coconut oil
- ➢ 1 egg
- ➢ Organic lemon peel
- ➢ 1 pinch cream of tartar
- ➢ 1 pinch baking soda
- ➢ Blueberries to taste

DIRECTIONS:

1. Make a workable mixture with all the ingredients.
2. Shape small balls and put one or more blueberries inside.
3. Bake at 355° F (180° C) for 15 minutes.

NUTRITION:

Calories 515 Carbs 37g Fat 8g Protein 37g

12) Cocoa and coconut cake with pumpkin cream

INGREDIENTS for 8 servings:

For the base:

- 1/2 cup coconut flour
- 2 tablespoons extra dark cocoa powder
- 1/2 cup water or plant milk or coffee
- 3 medium-sized eggs
- 1/4 cup margarine or butter
- 3/4 cup fresh cream
- 1/4 cup erythritol
- 1 level teaspoon baking powder
- 1/2 teaspoon baking soda
- For the pumpkin cream:
- 3/4 cup steamed pumpkin
- 1/4 cup fresh cream
- 1/2 cup Greek yogurt 5%
- 1/4 cup erythritol
- 1 tablespoon cocoa nibs or dark chocolate chips
- 1 sprinkle cocoa and turmeric

DIRECTIONS:

1. Mix the dry ingredients. Blend the eggs with the electric mixer until slightly whipped.
2. Add the erythritol and blend again. Melt the margarine in the microwave or in a small pan.
3. Add the cream and margarine, then blend. Add the dry ingredients and water, then blend again.
4. Pour the mixture into a small cake pan, greased and floured with bamboo fiber.
5. Bake in the preheated static oven at 345° F (175° C) for 25 minutes. In the meantime, blend the pumpkin and add the remaining ingredients for the cream.
6. Once the cake has cooled, cut into 3 layers and garnish with the pumpkin cream and cocoa nibs.

NUTRITION:

Calories 1057 Carbs 57g Fat 77g Protein 34g

13) Coconut and raspberry truffles

INGREDIENTS:

- 1 cup Greek yogurt 5%
- Frozen raspberries
- 1 generous tablespoon erythritol
- 1 cup shredded coconut
- Dark chocolate 85% to taste

DIRECTIONS:

1. Mix yogurt, coconut and erythritol. Take a bit of dough, add a raspberry in the middle and gently close the small ball.
2. Once finished, put in the freezer for a couple of hours.
3. Melt the chocolate. With the help of a toothpick, dip the balls in the chocolate.
4. Let them stand.

NUTRITION:

Calories 617 Carbs 28g Fat 48g Protein 18g

14) Coconut balls and truffles

INGREDIENTS:

1. 1 cup mascarpone cheese
2. 1 cup shredded coconut
3. 1/4 cup stevia
4. Bitter cocoa

DIRECTIONS:

1. Mix the mascarpone, coconut and stevia, and shape small balls.
2. Sprinkle with more coconut. Add some bitter cocoa to half of them to make truffles.
3. Let stand in the fridge for 2 hours.

NUTRITION:

Calories 711 Carbs 12g Fat 68g Protein 13g

15) Coconut pralines

INGREDIENTS:

- 1 cup ricotta cheese
- 1/4 cup sweetener
- 1 cup shredded coconut
- As many almonds as pralines
- 1/2 sachet vanillin (optional)

DIRECTIONS:

1. In a bowl, mix the ricotta cheese with the sweetener and the shredded coconut until you have a smooth and firm mixture.
2. Shape small balls and insert an almond (or toasted hazelnut) in each ball.
3. Dip them in the shredded coconut and let them stand in the fridge for at least 1 hour.

NUTRITION:

Calories 445 Carbs 18g Fat 29g Protein 29g

16) Coconut quindim
(Brazilian flan)

INGREDIENTS:

- 5 yolks
- 1/4 cup erythritol
- 1/4 cup shredded coconut
- 1/4 cup coconut milk

DIRECTIONS:

1. Beat the egg yolks with the sweetener.
2. Add the shredded coconut, milk and mix gently until smooth.
3. Fill the baking cups and bake in a bain-marie at 390° F (200° C) for about 25 minutes.

NUTRITION:

Calories 389 Carbs 4g Fat 35g Protein 15g

17) Cold lemon cake

INGREDIENTS:

For the base:

- 2 packages (3 1/2 ounce) gluten-free vanilla shortbread cookies by Tisanoreica
- 1/4 cup butter
- For the mousse:
- 1/4 cup fat-free, sugar-free Greek yogurt
- 1/2 cup water
- 1/4 ounce isinglass sheets
- 1/2 cup erythritol
- 1 lemon

For the gelee:

- 1/2 cup lemon juice
- 3/4 cup water
- 1/2 cup erythritol
- 1/4 ounce isinglass sheets
- Yellow coloring

DIRECTIONS:

1. For the base, melt the butter and mix it with the finely crumbled shortbread cookies.
2. With the base, fill the bottom of the mold and press with a spoon. Put in the fridge.
3. For the mousse, heat the water with the erythritol, then remove from heat and add the soaked and squeezed isinglass.
4. Pour the liquid over the yogurt and mix. Add the lemon juice and zest. Pour the mousse into the mold over the base. Place in the fridge.
5. For the gelee, heat the erythritol with the water and lemon juice, remove from heat and add the soaked and squeezed isinglass and coloring. Pour the gelee over the mousse and let stand in the fridge for at least 3-4 hours before enjoying.

NUTRITION:

Calories 756 Carbs 58g Fat 54g Protein 11g

18) Cream tart

INGREDIENTS:

For the base:

- ➤ 1 cup almond flour
- ➤ 1/4 cup Backprotein flour (or fine coconut flour)
- ➤ 1/4 cup melted butter
- ➤ 1 whole egg
- ➤ 1 teaspoon xanthan (or cream of tartar)
- ➤ 1/2 teaspoon baking powder
- ➤ 1/4 cup erythritol
- ➤ drops vanilla flavoring

For the filling:

- ➤ 1 cup Greek yogurt (or mascarpone cheese or cream)
- ➤ 1/4 cup erythritol (or lemon flavoring)
- ➤ 4/5 strawberries
- ➤ Chopped pistachios

DIRECTIONS:

1. In a bowl, mix the almond flour with the xanthan, baking powder and butter.
2. Add the egg lightly beaten with the flavoring and sweetener. Knead until you have a firm dough and let stand in the fridge for at least 2 hours (even overnight).
3. Roll out the dough between 2 sheets of baking paper, use a rolling pin to obtain a thickness of about 1/2 inch and cut out two equal shapes (for example two hearts).
4. Bake at 340° F (170° C) for 15/20 minutes. Once cold, decorate and fill as you prefer, for example with Greek yogurt flavored with lemon and strawberries.

NUTRITION:

Calories 1259 Carbs 58g Fat 89g Protein 55g

19) Creamy apple and yogurt cake

INGREDIENTS:

- ➤ 2 apples
- ➤ 1/2 cup yogurt (your favorite one)
- ➤ 1/4 cup erythritol (or 1 1/2 tablespoons honey or agave syrup)
- ➤ 1/2 cup gluten-free flour (such as peanut flour)
- ➤ 1 egg
- ➤ Organic lemon peel or cinnamon powder
- ➤ 1/2 tablespoon baking powder
- ➤ Peanut or cashew nut grains

DIRECTIONS:

1. Blend one of the two apples with the yogurt, egg, sweetener and lemon, then add the flour with baking powder.
2. Finally cut the other apple into cubes and put it into the mixture.
3. Pour the mixture into a 5-inch round mold lined with baking paper, sprinkle the surface with some peanut or cashew nut grains and bake at 355° F (180° C) for about 30 minutes. Serve immediately.

NUTRITION:

Calories 596 Carbs 69g Fat 14g Protein 49g

20) Crumble pie baked in air fryer

INGREDIENTS:

For the base:

- 4 tablespoons oatmeal
- 2 tablespoons chickpea flour
- 1 tablespoon coconut flour by Be a Fit Chef
- 2 tablespoons almond flour
- 2 teaspoons erythritol/sugar/stevia
- 1 egg
- 1/4 cup egg whites

For the filling:

- 1/4 cup ricotta cheese
- 1 tablespoon dark chocolate drops
- Sweetener to taste
- Berries to taste
- For the topping:
- Almonds
- Almond butter

DIRECTIONS:

1. In a bowl, beat roughly the egg and egg whites. After that, combine one half with the remaining ingredients for the base, then knead.
2. After getting a homogeneous dough, let stand in the fridge for a few minutes.
3. Line the mold with 3/4 of the dough and bake in the air fryer for 2 minutes at 320° F (160° C) or in the oven for 3/4 minutes at 355° F (180° C) in static mode.
4. Combine ricotta cheese, the other half of egg + egg white and chocolate drops adding a few drops of sweetener, then pour into the base. Put on top the berries and the remaining part of the dough crumbling it.
5. Bake in the air fryer for 8 minutes at 300° F (150° C) opening halfway through baking or in the oven for 30 minutes at 355° F (180° C) in static mode. Let stand in the fryer/oven for at least 40 minutes and then in the fridge for at least 2 hours. Garnish with almond butter and almonds.

NUTRITION:

Calories 530 Carbs 49g Fat 22g Protein 347g

21) Four-colored panna cotta

INGREDIENTS for 2-3 servings:

- 1 cup cream
- 1/2 cup mascarpone cheese
- 3 tablespoons erythritol
- Sweetener (Tic or stevia according to your own taste)
- 1/4 ounce isinglass
- Bitter cocoa

DIRECTIONS:

1. Put the isinglass in cold water, meanwhile put 1/2 cup of cream and erythritol in a pan and heat without bringing to a boil.
2. Turn off the heat, add the squeezed isinglass and stir.
3. In a separate bowl, blend with a hand mixer the mascarpone and the remaining cream until it becomes creamy.
4. Add the warmed cream continuing to mix and then add the sweetener to taste.
5. Divide the mixture into four equal parts, leaving one white and mixing the others with cocoa to obtain three different colors. Pour the mixtures in order from lightest to darkest in 2-3 molds or grass bowls in four steps.
6. Each time you pour a layer, keep it in the fridge for 10 minutes and then pour the other. After this, let stand in the fridge for 3-4 hours. To remove from the molds, place them in hot water and then serve on a plate.

NUTRITION:

Calories 556 Carbs 5g Fat 57g Protein 5g

22) Gorgonzola and hazelnut truffles

INGREDIENTS:

- ➤ 1/4 cup gorgonzola cheese
- ➤ 1/4 cup goat's milk cheese
- ➤ 1/2 cup mascarpone cheese
- ➤ Chopped hazelnuts
- ➤ Chopped walnuts

DIRECTIONS:

1. To make these very tasty truffles, you can use gorgonzola, goat's milk cheese and mascarpone cheese, or the creamy cheeses you like. Just mix them all together and shape small balls.
2. Then sprinkle them half with chopped hazelnuts and half with chopped walnuts. Place them in the fridge and take them out only when you want to serve them.

NUTRITION:

Calories 571 Carbs 9g Fat 50g Protein 22g

23) Hazelnut and pistachio cheesecake without cooking

INGREDIENTS:

For the base:

- ➤ 1/4 cup melted coconut oil
- ➤ 1 tablespoon bitter cocoa
- ➤ 1 tablespoon erythritol
- ➤ 1 cup hazelnut flour

For the cream:

- ➤ 1 cup lactose-free mascarpone cheese
- ➤ 3/4 cup lactose-free cream cheese
- ➤ 1 generous teaspoon pistachio cream by Revolution03

DIRECTIONS:

1. Mix all the ingredients for the base and transfer the mixture into the chosen mold (we recommend those in silicone).
2. Let stand for about an hour in the fridge. Mix all the ingredients for the cream and stuff. Garnish with pistachio cream and chopped pistachios.

NUTRITION:

Calories 1602 Carbs 39g Fat 152g Protein 20g

24) Keto almond and orange hearts

INGREDIENTS:

- ➤ 1 organic orange
- ➤ 1 egg and 1 egg white
- ➤ 1/4 cup erythritol
- ➤ 1 tablespoon orange peel powder
- ➤ 1/4 cup free-sugar almond milk
- ➤ 1/4 cup extra virgin olive oil
- ➤ 1 cup almond flour
- ➤ 1/3 cup almond slivers (also for decoration)
- ➤ 1/2 sachet baking powder

DIRECTIONS:

1. Blend the organic orange with the egg and egg white, erythritol and orange peel powder.
2. Add the milk, oil and baking powder and blend again.
3. Finally, add the almond flour and almond slivers.
4. Put the mixture in heart-shaped silicone molds and bake at 355° F (180° C) for 25 minutes.

NUTRITION:

Calories 1729 Carbs 64g Fat 137g Protein 59g

25) Keto bistro cake

INGREDIENTS:

➢ eggs
➢ 2/3 cup erythritol
➢ 1 1/2 cups butter (clarified if possible)
➢ 2 cups dark chocolate
➢ 1 pinch salt

DIRECTIONS:

1. Preheat the oven to 355° F (180° C).
2. Melt the chocolate together with the butter. Separate the yolks from the egg whites. Whip the egg whites until stiff and lightly beat the yolks with 1 pinch of salt.
3. Add the chocolate with the butter to the eggs, continuing to beat with an electric mixer. Gently incorporate the egg whites and mix.
4. Pour the mixture into a baking sheet lined with baking paper and bake for 25 minutes.

NUTRITION:

Calories 888 Carbs 9g Fat 84g Protein 26g

26) Keto blueberry cobbler

INGREDIENTS:

➢ 1 1/2 cups blueberries
➢ 1 1/2 cups almond flour
➢ 1/3 cup clarified butter
➢ 1 teaspoon cinnamon
➢ 2 heaped tablespoons erythritol
➢ Lemon juice
➢ 1 egg
➢ Vanilla flavoring

DIRECTIONS:

1. Preheat the oven to 375° F (190° C). In a baking sheet, put blueberries, cinnamon, 1 heaped tablespoon of erythritol and lemon juice. Stir and set aside.
2. In a bowl, mix almond flour, egg, melted butter, vanilla flavoring and knead with your hands.
3. Crumble the mixture over the blueberries. Top with the remaining erythritol and bake for 25 minutes.
4. Serve warm, maybe with whipped cream (if you really want to exaggerate).

NUTRITION:

Calories 1182 Carbs 68g Fat 82g Protein 68g

27) Keto Bundt cake

INGREDIENTS:

➢ 3 eggs
➢ 2 or 3 tablespoons erythritol
➢ 1/4 cup extra virgin olive oil
➢ 1/2 cup soy yogurt or almond yogurt
➢ Lemon peel
➢ 2 cups almond flour
➢ 1/2 tablespoon cream of tartar
➢ 1/2 tablespoon baking soda

DIRECTIONS:

1. Whip eggs with erythritol, add extra virgin olive oil and soy yogurt or almond yogurt, lemon peel, almond flour, cream of tartar and baking soda.
2. Bake in the oven at 355° F (180° C) for 30/35 minutes.

NUTRITION:

Calories 1325 Carbs 27g Fat 113g Protein 49g

28) Keto cannoli (Sicilian pastries)

INGREDIENTS:

- ➢ 2 cups almond flour
- ➢ 1/4 cup psyllium husk
- ➢ 1/4 cup erythritol
- ➢ Peel of 1 lemon or vanillin
- ➢ 1 tablespoon apple vinegar
- ➢ 1/4 cup water
- ➢ 1 egg
- ➢ 1 cup sheep ricotta
- ➢ 1/4 cup erythritol
- ➢ Chopped pistachios

DIRECTIONS:

1. Beat the egg with the water and vinegar, add the erythritol, then the almond flour, lemon peel and finally the psyllium husk.
2. Knead the dough, shape a ball and let stand in the fridge for 15 minutes.
3. After that, divide the dough into 8 balls that you will roll out between 2 sheets of baking paper with the help of a rolling pin. Roll the obtained disks on previously buttered cannoli molds and bake at 320° F (160° C) for 15 minutes.
4. Alternatively, this dough can also be fried. Stuff with the ricotta sweetened with erythritol and a sprinkle of chopped pistachios.

NUTRITION:

Calories 1303 Carbs 59g Fat 90g Protein 64g

29) Keto cassatelle (Sicilian half-moon pastries)

INGREDIENTS:

- ➢ 1 cup almond flour
- ➢ 1/3 cup erythritol
- ➢ 1 egg
- ➢ 2 tablespoons melted clarified butter
- ➢ 2 generous teaspoons xanthan gum
- ➢ Vanilla flavoring
- ➢ Goat's milk ricotta cheese to taste
- ➢ Extra dark chocolate 85%

DIRECTIONS:

1. Mix all the dry ingredients together, then add eggs and butter.
2. Knead to form a ball and let stand in the fridge for about 1 hour.
3. Meanwhile, prepare the filling by cutting the chocolate into small nuggets and mixing them together with the ricotta cheese.
4. Finely roll out the dough between 2 sheets of baking paper and cut out circles with a ring mold or a glass. Place a teaspoon of filling in the center, fold to form a half-moon and press the edges together.
5. Bake in the air fryer or in oil until golden brown.

NUTRITION:

Calories 764 Carbs 28g Fat 59g Protein 30g

30) Keto cinnamon dessert

INGREDIENTS for one serving:

- ➢ 1/4 cup Fage Greek yogurt 2% (choose whichever you prefer)
- ➢ 1/4 cup cinnamon muesli by Simply Keto
- ➢ 1 tablespoon red berry dessert by KFD Nutrition

DIRECTIONS:

1. Take a suitable glass, alternate layers of yogurt, red berry dessert and crunchy cinnamon muesli.
2. Let stand in the fridge for a few hours.

NUTRITION:

Calories 275 Carbs 12g Fat 20g Protein 12g

31) Keto coffee cake

INGREDIENTS for an 8-inch cake pan:

- ➢ 2 eggs
- ➢ 1/4 cup erythritol
- ➢ Vanilla
- ➢ 1 1/2 cups almond flour
- ➢ 3/4 cup sour cream
- ➢ 1/4 cup butter
- ➢ 1 teaspoon baking powder
- ➢ 3 teaspoons instant coffee
- ➢ 1 tablespoon cocoa nibs

DIRECTIONS:

1. Beat the whole eggs with the erythritol.
2. Mix all the other ingredients taking care to melt the butter.
3. Bake in the slow cooker or in the static oven at 355° F (180° C) for about 30 minutes.
4. Do the toothpick test.

NUTRITION:

Calories 954 Carbs 24g Fat 82g Protein 31g

32) Keto crêpe

INGREDIENTS:

- ➢ 1 egg
- ➢ 1 scoop Chokkino cocoa
- ➢ 1 tablespoon oat fiber (bamboo fiber is also fine)
- ➢ 2 tablespoons sugar-free almond milk
- ➢ Almond cream for filling by Revolution03

DIRECTIONS:

1. Beat the egg with the milk, cocoa and fiber.
2. Cook in a hot nonstick pan greased with coconut oil. Stuff with cream.

NUTRITION:

Calories 113 Carbs 4g Fat 7g Protein 7g

33) Keto cupcakes

INGREDIENTS:

- ➢ 1 cup almond flour
- ➢ 1/4 cup erythritol
- ➢ Vanillin or lemon peel
- ➢ 2 teaspoons baking powder
- ➢ 1/4 cup melted butter
- ➢ 1/4 cup sugar-free almond milk
- ➢ 2 eggs

DIRECTIONS:

1. Mix all the dry ingredients. In another bowl whisk together eggs, milk and melted butter.
2. Combine the two mixtures and pour into baking cups or a cupcake/muffin mold. Bake in the preheated static oven at 355° F (180° C) for 15 minutes.
3. You can enrich the cupcakes with whipped cream.

NUTRITION:

Calories 1083 Carbs 26g Fat 92g Protein 38g

34) Keto pandoro (Italian Christmas sweet bread)

INGREDIENTS:

- 3 cups almond flour
- 1/2 cup erythritol powder
- 1 cup hot water
- 1/4 cup butter
- 1/4 cup whey protein
- 1 tablespoon cream of tartar
- 1 tablespoon psyllium
- 1/4 cup sour cream
- 5 eggs
- 1/2 cup egg whites
- 1 teaspoon xanthan
- 1/2 tablespoon baking soda

DIRECTIONS:

1. Generously butter the appropriate mold. Mix the dry ingredients except the sweetener. Whip the egg whites and the yolks with the sweetener until stiff.
2. Mix the two whipped egg mixtures, the butter with the cream, and all the dry ingredients. Little by little, pour the mixture into the mold.
3. Bake in the static oven at 355° F (180° C) for 20 minutes and then at 320° F (160° C) for 1 hour. Keep the oven closed.
4. Let the pandoro cool before removing it from the mold and sprinkle with erythritol powder.

NUTRITION:

Calories 1585 Carbs 35g Fat 116g Protein 100g

35) Keto pastries with strawberry jam and peanut butter

INGREDIENTS:

- 2 1/2 cups almond flour
- 1/2 cup erythritol
- 2 1/2 teaspoons xanthan gum
- 1/4 cup almond milk
- 1/3 cup melted butter
- 1/2 tablespoon apple cider vinegar
- Keto strawberry jam
- Peanut butter

DIRECTIONS:

1. Mix all the dry ingredients in a bowl, add the melted butter and almond milk and knead with your hands until you have a dough like shortcrust pastry.
2. Wrap in baking paper and let stand in the freezer for 10 minutes.
3. Roll out between 2 sheets of baking paper, cut out rectangles (about 2 x 3 inch) and place half of them on a baking sheet.
4. Stuff with 1 teaspoon of peanut butter and 1 teaspoon of jam.
5. In the remaining half, make horizontal cuts, close the stuffed strips and seal with the tines of a fork. Brush with some almond milk and bake at 340° F (170° C) for 20/25 minutes.
6. Optional: Once cooled, decorate with icing prepared with powdered erythritol and water or even with dark chocolate.

NUTRITION:

Calories 686 Carbs 12g Fat 66g Protein 12g

36) Keto red velvet cake

INGREDIENTS:

- ➤ 1 1/2 cups almond flour
- ➤ 2 teaspoons bitter cocoa
- ➤ 2 teaspoons baking powder
- ➤ 1 teaspoon instant coffee (optional)
- ➤ 1 pinch salt
- ➤ 1/4 cup almond milk
- ➤ 3 eggs
- ➤ 1/2 cup erythritol
- ➤ 1 tablespoon white Greek yogurt
- ➤ Vanillin
- ➤ Red coloring

DIRECTIONS:

1. Mix with a whisk all the dry ingredients, add eggs, milk and Greek yogurt and finally the coloring.
2. Butter or cover the baking sheet with baking paper, pour the mixture and bake at 355° F (180° C) for 25/30 minutes. Stuff and decorate with whipped cream and a bit of imagination.

NUTRITION:

Calories 553 Carbs 15g Fat 39g Protein 35g

37) Lemon and blueberry cheesecake (gluten-free and egg-free)

INGREDIENTS:

For the base:
- ➤ 1 1/2 cups almond flour
- ➤ 1/2 cup rice flour
- ➤ 1/2 cup melted butter
- ➤ 1/4 cup sugar

For the cream:
- ➤ 1 cup Philadelphia cheese
- ➤ 1 cup mascarpone cheese
- ➤ 3/4 cup whipped cream
- ➤ 1 cup icing sugar
- ➤ 1/2 ounce gelatin sheets
- ➤ Juice of 2 lemons
- ➤ 1 cup blueberries
- ➤ 1 tablespoon corn starch

DIRECTIONS:

1. Mix all the ingredients to make the base, line a 7-inch cake pan and bake at 355° F (180° C) for 20 minutes. Prepare the blueberry jam by cooking the blueberries with the corn starch over low heat for about 15 minutes. Blend and let cool.
2. In a bowl, mix the Philadelphia, mascarpone and whipped cream with the icing sugar.
3. Divide into two bowls and in one of them simply add the lemon juice and half of the gelatin dissolved in a pan with a little water (do not pour it into the bowl when it is boiling, otherwise it will make lumps).
4. In the other half of the mixture, add two or three tablespoons of blueberry jam and the remaining melted and warmed gelatin.
5. On the cooled base, pour the lemon mixture. Place in the freezer for half an hour and then pour in the blueberry mixture. Keep in the freezer for another half an hour and then top the cake with the remaining jam. Decorate with fresh blueberries and store in the freezer. Take it out of the freezer an hour or so before serving.

NUTRITION:

Calories 1692 Carbs 109g Fat 129g Protein 24g

38) Lemon bonbon with raspberry cream

INGREDIENTS for three 3-inch bonbons:

➢ For the base:
➢ 2 tablespoons lemon-flavored oats
➢ 2 tablespoons soy flour
➢ 2 tablespoons neutral oat flour
➢ 1/4 cup lemon juice and pulp
➢ Grated lemon peel
➢ 1/2 tablespoon Bolero Lemon Pie flavoring
➢ 1/2 tablespoon instant yeast
➢ 1/4 cup white Greek yogurt
➢ 1/3 cup egg whites
➢ For the cream:
➢ 3/4 cup raspberries
➢ 1/2 tablespoon bamboo flour
➢ 1 teaspoon erythritol

DIRECTIONS:

1. Mix with a whisk all the powders for the bonbons and add the yogurt and then the juice and egg whites.
2. Let stand and in the meantime prepare the raspberry cream by cooking them on a nonstick pan and letting them dry a bit. Then add the sweetener and bamboo flour.
3. Pour more than half of the mixture into 3-inch half sphere-shaped silicone molds. Bake in the microwave at 750 W for 2 minutes with a small cup of water on the turntable plate.
4. After that, take them out of the microwave and with a teaspoon create a hole in the middle of each bonbon. Pour the raspberry cream, cover with more dough and bake in the microwave for another 1/2 minute.
5. Let cool and enjoy cold.

NUTRITION:

Calories 275 Carbs 39g Fat 4g Protein 21g

39) Low carb bicolor protein cake

INGREDIENTS for an 8 x 8-in cake pan:

➢ 3 organic eggs
➢ 1 mashed ripe banana
➢ 1 tablespoon ghee or coconut oil
➢ 1/2 cup sugar-free Greek yogurt
➢ 1/2 cup coconut flour
➢ 1/2 cup almond flour
➢ 1 sachet baking powder
➢ 1 pinch Himalayan salt
➢ 2 tablespoons bitter cocoa
➢ 1 tablespoon stevia 1:8

DIRECTIONS:

1. Separate the yolks from the egg whites and beat the latter until stiff.
2. Separately, mash the banana until it becomes a puree, add the yolks, ghee (or coconut oil) and blend or mix with a whisk. Once you have a soft cream, add the yogurt and the "fat flours", salt and baking powder.
3. Finally add the egg whites beaten until stiff, mixing from the bottom up.
4. At this point, separate the mixture into two bowls. In one add the bitter cocoa and stevia.
5. Preheat the oven to 355° F (180° C). Line a cake pan with baking paper and pour first the white mixture and then the cocoa mixture, trying not to mix them.
6. Bake in the static oven for about 45 minutes (the time varies from oven to oven, always do the toothpick test!). Once cooled, you can sprinkle with grated coconut (optional).
7. This cake can be frozen by cutting slices and wrapping them in plastic wrap. To thaw, simply remove from the freezer and place in the fridge in the evening to be ready for breakfast the next day.

NUTRITION:

Calories 908 Carbs 56g Fat 55g Protein 47g

40) Low carb & keto marble cake

INGREDIENTS for a 16-serving cake:

For the base:

- ➢ 1 cup low carb coconut flour
- ➢ 1/4 cup almond or hazelnut flour
- ➢ 3 tablespoons potato fiber
- ➢ 2/3 cup butter or coconut oil
- ➢ medium-sized eggs
- ➢ 1 cup erythritol + stevia (Sukrin) mixture
- ➢ 1 sachet baking powder
- ➢ 2 tablespoons low fat cocoa

For the icing:

- ➢ 1 1/2 tablespoons coconut oil
- ➢ 1/2 cup sugar-free dark chocolate

DIRECTIONS:

1. Preheat the fan oven to 345° F (175° C). Prepare a 10-inch cake mold and sprinkle it with oil (even if it is a nonstick or silicone mold).
2. Beat the coconut oil softened with the sweetener and then add the eggs one at a time.
3. Add the almond or hazelnut flour, coconut flour, potato fiber and baking powder and mix to obtain a smooth dough.
4. Divide the mixture into two parts. Put one part in the mold and add the cocoa to the other, mix and then pour the dark mixture over the light one.
5. Mix just enough to get the marble effect. Bake for 50-60 minutes. Let cool for at least 10 minutes before removing the cake from the mold.
6. For the icing, melt the coconut oil and chocolate in the microwave and mix until smooth. Brush the top of the cooled cake and then place in the fridge so that the icing solidifies.

NUTRITION:

Calories 1054 Carbs 55g Fat 79g Protein 31g

41) Low carb ricotta cake

INGREDIENTS:

For the shortcrust pastry:

- ➢ 3/4 cup RevoMix Pasta flour by Revolution03
- ➢ 3/4 cup RevoMix Cake flour by Revolution03
- ➢ 1/4 cup erythritol
- ➢ 1/2 cup lactose-free butter
- ➢ 2 eggs
- ➢ 1/2 sachet baking powder
- ➢ Vanilla essence
- ➢ Lemon peel to taste
- ➢ For the ricotta cream:
- ➢ 3/4 cup goat's milk ricotta cheese
- ➢ 1/4 cup pistachio flour
- ➢ 2 tablespoons erythritol
- ➢ chopped pistachios
- ➢ 2 tablespoons Pistacchio Zero cream by Revolution03
- ➢ 1 egg

DIRECTIONS:

1. Reduce erythritol and lemon peel to powder.
2. Add cold butter, flour mixture, baking powder, vanilla essence and eggs in a kneader and knead for a few minutes.
3. Shape a loaf and let stand in the fridge. After about an hour, roll out the shortcrust pastry to be filled.
4. Blend the ingredients for the cream all together and fill the previous made shortcrust pastry.
5. Decorate and bake at 340° F (170° C) for 40 minutes.

NUTRITION:

Calories 1092 Carbs 50g Fat 67g Protein 42g

42) Mini protein magnums

INGREDIENTS:

- ➢ For 4 mini magnums:
- ➢ 1/4 cup vanilla-flavored protein powder
- ➢ 1 cup thick coconut milk
- ➢ 1 tablespoon erythritol
- ➢ Vanilla flavoring (optional)
- ➢ Extra dark chocolate 85%
- ➢ Shredded coconut

DIRECTIONS:

1. Blend the protein, milk, erythritol and flavoring.
2. Transfer the mixture into silicone ice cream molds.
3. Let stand in the freezer overnight. For the icing, melt the chocolate, dip the ice cream and place it on a sheet of aluminum foil.
4. Add the coconut and let cool.

NUTRITION:

Calories 393 Carbs 11g Fat 25g Protein 32g

43) Pina colada chia pudding

INGREDIENTS for 2 servings:

- ➢ 1/2 cup pineapple
- ➢ 1/4 cup shredded coconut
- ➢ 1/4 cup chia seeds
- ➢ 1 cup coconut cream (milk)
- ➢ 2-3 drops coconut-flavored sweetener (optional)

DIRECTIONS:

1. Blend the pineapple together with the coconut milk.
2. Add the shredded coconut, sweetener and chia seeds.
3. Mix, let stand for a couple of hours and enjoy.

NUTRITION:

Calories 172 Carbs 12g Fat 13g Protein 3g

44) Red fruit panna cotta (Italian dessert of sweetened cream)

INGREDIENTS:

- ➢ 2 cups fresh cream
- ➢ 1/2 ounce gelatin sheets
- ➢ 1/4 cup frozen wild berries
- ➢ 1/4 cup erythritol

DIRECTIONS:

1. Place the gelatin sheets in cold water. Heat the cream, add most of the erythritol and a little vanilla extract. In the meantime, put in a pan the wild berries with the remaining erythritol and squeeze 1/2 lemon. Cook for 10 minutes.
2. Add almost all the softened gelatin sheets (set aside a small piece for the topping) to the hot cream and bring to a boil.
3. Remove from heat and divide into 4/6 small bowls. Place them in the fridge.
4. Blend the berries with a little bit of cream and bring back on the stove.
5. Add the piece of gelatin sheet and let melt. When the cream has cooled, add the topping and put in the fridge.

NUTRITION:

Calories 763 Carbs 11g Fat 78g Protein 6g

45) Ricotta and chocolate moist cake

INGREDIENTS:

For the base:

- ➢ 1 egg
- ➢ 2 teaspoons stevia
- ➢ 1/2 cup ricotta cheese
- ➢ 1/2 cup chocolate oatmeal
- ➢ 1 tablespoon extra dark chocolate
- ➢ 1 teaspoon baking powder
- ➢ 1 tablespoon free-sugar milk

For the topping:

- ➢ 1 tablespoon Ciobar Zero
- ➢ Water

DIRECTIONS:

1. Mix the ingredients and bake in the static oven at 355° F (180° C) for 35 minutes.
2. Mix the Ciobar with the water to create the cream.
3. Let stand in the fridge for half an hour and enjoy!

NUTRITION:

Calories 245 Carbs 23g Fat 13g Protein 10g

46) Rum truffles

INGREDIENTS for 16 truffles:

- ➢ 1/3 cup lactose-free ricotta cheese
- ➢ 1/4 cup butter
- ➢ 1/2 cup almonds reduced to flour
- ➢ 1 teaspoon stevia (or tic/erythritol to taste)
- ➢ A few drops rum flavoring
- ➢ Cinnamon (optional)
- ➢ Cocoa to taste
- ➢ Hazelnuts or almonds to taste

DIRECTIONS:

1. Melt the butter. Mix all the ingredients together and let cool in the fridge.
2. Form small balls putting inside a hazelnut or almond.
3. Dip in bitter cocoa and put back in the fridge. Serve cold.
4. Tip: to coat the truffles with cocoa, put 1 tablespoon of cocoa in a bag along with the balls and shake.

NUTRITION:

Calories 965 Carbs 22g Fat 83g Protein 34g

47) Pistachio cake

INGREDIENTS:

- ➢ 1 cup RevoMix Cake flour by Revolution03
- ➢ 1/4 cup pistachio flour
- ➢ 1 sachet instant yeast
- ➢ 3 eggs
- ➢ 1/2 cup melted ghee
- ➢ 1/4 cup Greek yogurt

DIRECTIONS:

1. Mix the dry ingredients. Mix the liquid ingredients and then blend them together with the dry ones.
2. Pour the mixture into an 8-inch cake pan and bake at 340° F (170° C) for about 30 minutes. Do the toothpick test.
3. For the filling you can use whipped cream, Pistacchio Zero cream and chopped pistachios.

NUTRITION:

Calories 1125 Carbs 93g Fat 68g Protein 34g

48) Sachertorte cake

INGREDIENTS:

- 1 cup RevoMix Cake flour by Revolution03
- 1/2 cup bitter cocoa
- 1 sachet baking powder
- 4 eggs
- 1/2 cup melted coconut oil
- 1/2 cup cream

DIRECTIONS:

1. Mix the dry ingredients. Beat the eggs, add the cream and coconut oil, then add the dry ingredients.
2. If needed, add sweetener to taste.
3. Pour the mixture into a buttered 8-inch cake pan.
4. Bake at 340° F (170° C) for about 40 minutes. For the filling, you can use for example homemade raspberry jam and ganache.

NUTRITION:

Calories 1209 Carbs 87g Fat 78g Protein 40g

49) Sponge cake with cream and cherry compote

INGREDIENTS:

For the base:

- 2 cups almond flour
- 1/2 cup erythritol
- 4 eggs
- 1 teaspoon baking powder
- 1/4 cup very cold water

For the cream:

- 1/2 cup whipped cream
- 1/4 cup Greek yogurt
- 1/4 cup Philadelphia cheese
- Lemon peel
- Sweetener to taste
- A few drops rum flavoring
- For the cherry compote:
- 20 cherries
- Powdered erythritol to taste
- Lemon peel and juice to taste

DIRECTIONS:

1. Using a whisk, beat the eggs with the erythritol.
2. Add the flour, water and baking powder and continue to mix until all ingredients are well combined.
3. Pour the mixture in a 7 inch cake pan. Bake at 355° F (180° C) for 20 minutes. Let cool in the oven.
4. For the cream compote, blend everything and set aside.
5. For the cherry compote, blend everything and set aside.
6. Now compose the cake. Take the sponge cake and hollow it out leaving a 1 inch edge. Be careful not to pierce the bottom. Make a syrup of coconut milk, erythritol and rum drops to moisten the sponge cake.
7. Pour a layer of cream, then pour the cherry compote.
8. Finally, decorate with the remaining cream. Let stand in the fridge for at least a couple of hours before serving.

NUTRITION:

Calories 1231 Carbs 55g Fat 84g Protein 62g

50) Stracciatella cake

INGREDIENTS for 1 serving:

- 2 1/2 tablespoons almond flour
- 1 tablespoon erythritol
- 1 teaspoon baking powder
- 1 egg
- 1/4 cup fresh ricotta cheese
- 1/4 cup vanilla skyr
- 1 tablespoon dark chocolate 90%

DIRECTIONS:

1. Mix everything adding chopped dark chocolate at the end and pour into a bowl, lightly greased with coconut oil.
2. Cook in a bain-marie for about 20 minutes.
3. Once warmed, sprinkle with more chopped dark chocolate.

NUTRITION:

Calories 820 Carbs 36g Fat 59g Protein 37g

51) Strawberry donuts

INGREDIENTS:

For the donuts:

- ➢ 1 cup almond flour
- ➢ 1/4 cup creamy cheese
- ➢ 1 egg
- ➢ 1/4 cup erythritol
- ➢ 1 1/2 tablespoons melted butter
- ➢ Vanillin or lemon peel
- ➢ 1 teaspoon baking powder
- ➢ 1 pinch salt
- ➢ 1 tablespoon sugar-free almond milk

For the strawberry coulis:

- ➢ 1/2 cup strawberries
- ➢ Juice and peel of 1 lemon
- ➢ 1/4 cup erythritol

DIRECTIONS:

1. For the strawberry coulis, put in a pan all the ingredients and cook for just 5 minutes. After that, blend and let cool.
2. For the donuts, mix all the ingredients and blend with the electric mixer until smooth.
3. Butter a donut or muffin mold and pour the mixture.
4. Bake in the preheated oven at 320° F (160° C) for 15-20 minutes, until golden brown on the surface.
5. Before serving, pour your now cold coulis over the donuts.

NUTRITION:

Calories 958 Carbs 42g Fat 72g Protein 37g

52) Tiramisu roll

INGREDIENTS:

- ➢ 3 eggs
- ➢ 1/4 cup erythritol
- ➢ 1/4 cup coconut flour
- ➢ Vanilla flavoring
- ➢ 1/2 teaspoon cream of tartar
- ➢ 1 cup mascarpone cheese
- ➢ 1 espresso
- ➢ Bitter cocoa powder
- ➢ Almond milk to taste
- ➢ Liquid sweetener for the cream (optional)

DIRECTIONS:

1. Brew the espresso and set aside. Separate the yolks from the egg whites.
2. Whip the egg whites until stiff, add the yolks previously mixed with erythritol and finally add the coconut flour and cream of tartar.
3. Transfer the mixture into a baking sheet covered with baking paper and bake for about 12 minutes at 340° F (170° C). Check the browning.
4. Let cool and in the meantime prepare the cream. Blend the mascarpone cheese, vanilla flavoring, sweetener and almond milk (the cream should be soft but firm).
5. With a pastry brush, wet the base with the cold expresso, add the mascarpone cream and roll it up with the help of the baking paper. Close the roll with aluminum foil and let stand in the fridge for at least 3 hours. Sprinkle with cocoa before serving.

NUTRITION:

Calories 732 Carbs 21g Fat 60g Protein 27g

53) Vanilla and pomegranate pudding (vegan and gluten-free)

INGREDIENTS for 3 people:

For the pudding:

- ➢ 1 tablespoon corn flour
- ➢ 1/2 teaspoon agar-agar
- ➢ 3 tablespoons sweetener or erythritol
- ➢ 1 teaspoon vanilla powder
- ➢ 1 cup plant milk of your choice
- ➢ 1/2 cup cashews, soaked in hot water for one hour

For the pomegranate topping:

- ➢ 1/2 cup pomegranate juice
- ➢ 1 teaspoon corn flour
- ➢ 1/2 teaspoon agar-agar

DIRECTIONS:

1. Blend all the ingredients for the topping and then cook over very low heat for 10 minutes.
2. Pour into glasses and let cool completely.
3. Prepare the topping by combining the ingredients and cooking over low heat for about 5 minutes.
4. Pour the cooled topping over the vanilla pudding and let stand in the fridge.

NUTRITION:

Calories 239 Carbs 35g Fat 1g Protein 23g

54) Watermelon ice pop with dark chocolate chips

INGREDIENTS:

- ➢ 1 cup watermelon pulp
- ➢ 1/2 cup coconut milk
- ➢ 1 tablespoon Philadelphia cheese
- ➢ Juice of 1/2 lemon
- ➢ Sweetener to taste
- ➢ Dark chocolate chips

DIRECTIONS:

1. Remove the seeds from the watermelon pulp, then put the ingredients in a blender (except chocolate) and blend everything.
2. Add some chocolate chips and pour into molds.
3. Cut out the base with some watermelon to fit the shape of your molds, make a cut in the middle to insert the stick, then use it as a cap.
4. Let stand in the freezer, overnight if possible. Finally remove the ice pops from the molds and top with more dark chocolate chips.

NUTRITION:

Calories 284 Carbs 48g Fat 9g Protein 2g

55) Wild berry ice cream

INGREDIENTS:

- ➢ 2 cups wild berry mix
- ➢ 2 cups sugar-free fresh cream
- ➢ 3/4 cup erythritol
- ➢ Juice and peel of 1 lemon

DIRECTIONS:

1. Cook the berries with erythritol, juice and lemon peel in a small pan over low heat for 5 minutes. Blend and let cool.
2. With the electric mixer, lightly whip the cream and add it to the now cold wild berry compote.
3. Place it in a freezer container and let stand for at least 2 hours.
4. To enjoy your wild berry ice cream at its best, take it out of the freezer 30 minutes before serving it.

NUTRITION:

Calories 195 Carbs 37g Fat 4g Protein 3g

56) Yule log (Christmas cake)

INGREDIENTS:

For the base:
- ➢ 1 cup egg whites
- ➢ 1/2 cup bitter cocoa powder
- ➢ Hazelnut flavoring
- ➢ 1/4 cup erythritol
- ➢ 1 cup mascarpone cheese
- ➢ 1/4 cup Greek yogurt
- ➢ 1/4 cup dark chocolate 99%

For garnish:
- ➢ 1 cup sugar-free cream
- ➢ 1 tablespoon erythritol (you can add more according to your taste)
- ➢ 1 tablespoon bitter cocoa powder
- ➢ Chopped hazelnuts or pistachios

DIRECTIONS:

1. In a blender, mix the egg whites with the bitter cocoa powder and flavoring (you can also sweeten with stevia, tic or erythritol).
2. Blend for a few seconds to make the mixture smooth, grease with coconut oil a nonstick pan and pour the mixture forming a large crêpe.
3. Cook with the lid on for a few minutes and then carefully turn over and cook for a few more minutes.
4. While the crêpe is cooling, whip the Greek yogurt with the erythritol and mascarpone with an electric mixer, then add the dark chocolate pieces.
5. Stuff the crêpe and roll it. Let stand in the fridge for at least 1 hour before cutting off one end to form the branch of the log. Whip the cream with the erythritol and cocoa and decorate the log with chopped hazelnuts or pistachios.

NUTRITION:

Calories 418 Carbs 10g Fat 24g Protein 39g

57) Zebra cake

INGREDIENTS:

- ➢ 1/4 cup coconut oil or extra virgin olive oil
- ➢ 1/4 cup coconut yogurt
- ➢ 1 cup almond flour
- ➢ 1/4 cup coconut flour
- ➢ 3 eggs
- ➢ 2 tablespoons erythritol
- ➢ Organic lemon peel
- ➢ Blueberry powder to taste
- ➢ 1/2 teaspoon baking soda + 1/2 teaspoon cream of tartar

DIRECTIONS:

1. Whip the eggs with the erythritol, add the oil, yogurt and lemon peel.
2. Finally add the dry ingredients continuing with the electric mixer.
3. Divide the dough in two parts and add the blueberry powder or cocoa powder.
4. Fill a 7 inch cake pan alternating the two mixtures. Bake at 355° F (180° C) for 30 minutes.

NUTRITION:

Calories 1081 Carbs 36g Fat 85g Protein 44g

11
DINNER RECIPES

1) Avocado bread

INGREDIENTS:

- 2 avocados
- 1/2 cup Parmesan cheese
- 2 eggs
- Salt
- Pepper
- Lemon juice
- Mixed seeds to taste

DIRECTIONS:

1. Mash the avocado flesh with a fork. Add eggs, salt, pepper and grated Parmesan cheese.
2. In a baking sheet covered with baking paper, shape some "mounds" with the help of a spoon.
3. Add the mixed seeds and bake for 35 minutes at 355° F (180° C) checking the browning.
4. Let cool and stuff as you prefer.

NUTRITION:

Calories 934 Carbs 7g Fat 84g Protein 39g

2) Avocado, frankfurter sausage and hazelnuts

INGREDIENTS:

- 1 avocado
- 4 frankfurter sausages
- Lactose-free Philadelphia cheese
- 1 handful chopped hazelnuts
- Extra virgin olive oil
- Salt and pepper
- Lemon juice to taste

DIRECTIONS:

1. Cut the sausages in half and cook them in a pan. Cut the avocado in half.
2. Put one half in a blender with extra virgin olive oil, salt, pepper and Philadelphia, blend and set aside.
3. Slice the other half and add lemon juice immediately so it doesn't blacken.
4. Serve the sausages with the sliced avocado and hazelnuts.
5. Put the previously prepared avocado cream in a plastic bag, cut the corner with the help of the scissors and decorate the plate.

NUTRITION:

Calories 889 Carbs 11g Fat 83g Protein 25g

3) Cooked ham and smoked scamorza roll

INGREDIENTS:

- ➢ 1/4 cup julienned mozzarella cheese
- ➢ 1/4 cup cream cheese
- ➢ 1 generous tablespoon almond flour
- ➢ 1 1/2 tablespoons linseed flour
- ➢ 1 tablespoon psyllium husk
- ➢ 1 tablespoon oil
- ➢ 1 pinch salt

DIRECTIONS:

1. Preheat the oven to 390° F (200° C). In a bowl, put the cheeses and let them melt completely in the microwave.
2. Add the flours, oil and salt and knead with your hands.
3. Roll out the dough between 2 sheets of baking paper (not too thin).
4. Stuff with 3 slices of cooked ham and 3 slices of smoked scamorza.
5. Roll up and close the sides. Sprinkle with sesame and poppy seeds. Bake for 15 minutes, let cool and enjoy.

NUTRITION:

Calories 276 Carbs 15g Fat 18g Protein 14g

4) Egg white roll

INGREDIENTS:

- ➢ 1/2 cup egg whites
- ➢ 1/2 grated zucchini
- ➢ Philadelphia
- ➢ Turkey breast
- ➢ Salt and pepper to taste

DIRECTIONS:

1. Whip the egg whites with salt and pepper, add the grated zucchini (which you have previously squeezed), mix and pour the mixture on the baking sheet lined with baking paper, not too thick.
2. Bake at 390° F (200° C) for 10/15 minutes.
3. Once cold, spread the Philadelphia and cover with slices of turkey breast, then roll, cut into rounds and enjoy.

NUTRITION:

Calories 256 Carbs 10g Fat 9g Protein 33g

5) Flaxseed baguette

INGREDIENTS:

- ➢ 1/3 cup flaxseed flour
- ➢ 1 tablespoon psyllium husk
- ➢ 1 sachet instant yeast
- ➢ Salt
- ➢ 1/4 cup hot water
- ➢ 1 teaspoon extra virgin olive oil
- ➢ 1/4 cup egg whites

DIRECTIONS:

1. Mix everything together in a bowl with a spoon. Let stand for 10 minutes.
2. Shape the baguettes with wet hands. Bake at 355° F (180° C) for 35 minutes.
3. Let cool and stuff as you like, for example with cheddar salad and baked pork.

NUTRITION:

Calories 282 Carbs 24g Fat 13g Protein 17g

6) Gorgonzola cheese and pistachio dumpling

INGREDIENTS:

- 2 eggs
- 1/4 cup gorgonzola cheese
- Chopped pistachios

DIRECTIONS:

1. Beat the eggs. Cook the omelet in a hot nonstick pan.
2. Stuff with 3/4 of the gorgonzola cheese and close the dumpling.
3. Pour the remaining melted gorgonzola and add the chopped pistachios.

NUTRITION:

Calories 259 Carbs 2g Fat 19g Protein 20g

7) Keto focaccia bread

INGREDIENTS:

- 1/2 cup coconut flour
- 1/4 cup flaxseed flour by Bulk
- 3 whole eggs
- 3/4 cups egg whites
- 5 tablespoons extra virgin olive oil
- 1/2 tablespoon instant yeast
- 1/2 cup natural water
- 1/2 teaspoon pink salt
- Provençal herbs or spices to taste

DIRECTIONS:

1. Mix the eggs and egg whites in a kneader until you get a frothy cream.
2. Add the remaining ingredients slowly, mixing with the kneader (or electric mixer) until you get a smooth dough.
3. Preheat the static oven to 355° F (180° C) and line with baking paper an 8 x 10-in baking sheet. Pour the mixture and level it.
4. Season like a normal focaccia bread and bake for about 35 minutes.

NUTRITION:

Calories 1221 Carbs 31g Fat 100g Protein 31g

8) Keto focaccia with pesto, bacon, walnuts and dried tomatoes

INGREDIENTS:

- 1 cup egg whites
- 3/4 cup almond flour
- 1/4 cup golden flaxseed flour
- 1 cup grated cheese
- Olive oil
- Salt
- Pepper
- Coarse salt
- Rosemary
- Bacon, walnuts, dried tomatoes, pesto to taste

DIRECTIONS:

1. Mix the flours, egg whites, cheese and oil.
2. Arrange evenly in a 9-inch baking sheet lined with baking paper and garnish with pesto, walnuts, diced bacon, dried tomatoes, rosemary and a sprinkle of coarse salt.
3. Bake in the fan oven at 390° F (200° C) for 20/25 minutes.

NUTRITION:

Calories 1443 Carbs 32g Fat 56g Protein 120g

9) Keto hot dog

INGREDIENTS for 2:

- ➢ 1/4 cup cream cheese
- ➢ 1/3 cup grated mozzarella cheese
- ➢ 1/3 cup almond flour
- ➢ 1/2 teaspoon yeast
- ➢ Sausages

DIRECTIONS:

1. Mix the cheeses and melt them in the microwave or in a bain-marie, add the almond flour and baking powder.
2. Once you have a homogeneous dough, divide it into two loaves and roll them out with your hands.
3. Wrap the dough around the sausages that you have previously cut on the ends.
4. Bake at 390° F (200° C) for about 10 minutcs.

NUTRITION:

Calories 646 Carbs 18g Fat 44g Protein 45g

10) Keto pizza

INGREDIENTS for 2 pizzas:

For the base:

- ➢ 1 cup egg whites
- ➢ 3/4 cup almond flour
- ➢ 1/4 cup golden linseed flour
- ➢ 1 cup grated Parmesan cheese
- ➢ 1 pinch salt

For the filling:

- ➢ 1 cup mozzarella cheese
- ➢ 1 cup spiralized zucchini
- ➢ 1 cup olives
- ➢ 1/2 cup sun-dried tomatoes

DIRECTIONS:

1. Mix all the ingredients for the base and divide the mixture in two.
2. Spread in a baking sheet with a spatula. Bake in the hot oven (fan mode) at 390° F (200° C) for 5 minutes.
3. Then turn upside down and stuff as you prefer.
4. Bake for another 15-20 minutes in the hot oven (fan mode) at 390° F (200° C).

NUTRITION:

Calories 1557 Carbs 36g Fat 109g Protein 106g

11) Keto pretzel

(German bread)

INGREDIENTS:

- ➢ 1 sachet brewer's yeast
- ➢ 1 teaspoon inulin
- ➢ 4 tablespoons hot water (not boiling)
- ➢ 2 cups almond flour
- ➢ 1 cup Galbanino cheese
- ➢ 1/2 cup Philadelphia cheese
- ➢ 2 eggs at room temperature
- ➢ Whole coarse salt
- ➢ 1 egg yolk

DIRECTIONS:

1. First melt the yeast with the inulin in the water and set the mixture aside until its volume doubles.
2. Melt the cheeses in the microwave or in a bain-marie.
3. Add the almond flour to the cheeses, then add the eggs. Knead the dough with your hands until smooth.
4. Divide the dough into 6-8 loaves that you will roll out with your hands to obtain the classic pretzel shape.
5. Brush with lightly beaten egg yolk and sprinkle with whole coarse salt (it's not as salty as sea salt and is rich in minerals).
6. Bake in the preheated oven at 390° F (200° C) for about 15 minutes.

NUTRITION:

Calories 1951 Carbs 55g Fat 151g Protein 94g

12) Keto sandwich

INGREDIENTS for 1 large sandwich:

- 1/2 cup almond flour
- 1 teaspoon psyllium
- 2 tablespoons coconut oil, melted
- 2 egg whites
- 1 teaspoon yeast
- Salt
- (1/2 cup erythritol for the sweet version)

DIRECTIONS:

1. Mix all the dry ingredients and add the egg whites mixed with coconut oil.
2. Roll out the dough between 2 sheets of baking paper and give it a square shape.
3. Bake in the oven at 355° F (180° C) for 15 minutes. Stuff as you prefer.

NUTRITION:

Calories 588 Carbs 19g Fat 48g Protein 19g

13) Keto sofficini

(Italian cheese turnovers)

INGREDIENTS for 3 sofficini:

- 1 cup cheese flakes
- 1 egg
- 2 tablespoons almond flour
- 2 tablespoons Parmesan cheese
- 3 teaspoons psyllium
- 1/2 teaspoon yeast
- Salt, pepper, marjoram
- 1/2 cup water

DIRECTIONS:

1. Put the cheese flakes, egg and water in a blender.
2. Blend everything, then add the remaining ingredients until thick.
3. Divide the mixture into three and cook in a heated pan greased with oil, as if you were going to make pancakes.
4. You'll see that the mixture slowly melts and puffs up.
5. Cook over low heat for about 10 minutes, until a crust forms on the bottom.

6. With the help of a plate, turn and then put back into the pan. Let the crust form, put back into the pan and stuff as you prefer, for example with bacon and grated Emmenthal cheese.
7. Fold and finally put back into the pan to melt the cheese.

NUTRITION:

Calories 756 Carbs 29g Fat 52g Protein 43g

14) Keto toast

INGREDIENTS:

- 1 cup egg whites
- 5 tablespoons sunflower seeds
- 2 tablespoons flax seeds
- 2 tablespoons sesame seeds
- Salt and garlic powder

DIRECTIONS:

1. Reduce the seeds to flour, add the egg whites and put the dough into square molds.
2. Bake in the oven at 355° F (180° C) for 20/25 minutes.
3. Stuff as you prefer, for example with bresaola, Parmesan shavings, cashews, poppy seeds and olive oil.

NUTRITION:

Calories 279 Carbs 8g Fat 13g Protein 32g

15) Keto wrap

INGREDIENTS for 2 people:

- ➤ 1 cup egg whites
- ➤ 1 tablespoon psyllium
- ➤ 1/2 cup mixed seed flour (flax, pumpkin, sesame)
- ➤ Salt

DIRECTIONS:

1. Mix all the ingredients with a whisk (avoid creating lumps).
2. Using a spatula, spread the dough directly into a hot nonstick pan.
3. Cook for a couple of minutes per side. When the base detaches easily from the pan, turn and finish cooking.
4. Stuff as you prefer (for example with cooked ham, 1 teaspoon of spicy mayonnaise, lettuce and cheese), then roll.

NUTRITION:

Calories 546 Carbs 17g Fat 34g Protein 42g

16) Low carb hamburger

INGREDIENTS for 1 hamburger:

- ➤ 2/3 cup RevoMix Pizza flour by Revolution03
- ➤ 1/4 cup water
- ➤ 1/2 tablespoon clarified butter (for seasoning, optional) or oil
- ➤ Milk
- ➤ Seeds

DIRECTIONS:

1. Mix the flour, water and butter or oil. Let stand for 1/2 hour, form a ball, brush with a little milk (even plant milk) and decorate with seeds.
2. Bake in the air fryer or oven at 355° F (180° C) for 15 minutes.
3. Cut and stuff as you prefer, for example with some filleted (lean) pork loin and caramelized onions.

NUTRITION:

Calories 217 Carbs 17g Fat 10g Protein 14g

17) Low carb piadina (stuffed flatbread)

INGREDIENTS:

- ➤ 1/4 cup flaxseed flour
- ➤ 2 1/2 tablespoons coconut flour
- ➤ 1/2 tablespoon psyllium powder
- ➤ 1/2 teaspoon baking soda
- ➤ 1 teaspoon apple cider vinegar
- ➤ 1/2 cup warm water

DIRECTIONS:

1. Put warm water and vinegar in a bowl.
2. Separately, sift the remaining ingredients and then add them to the water while continuing to mix.
3. Once amalgamated, gently knead for a few minutes. Roll out with a rolling pin to obtain the thickness of the classic piadina.
4. Heat a suitable pan and cook the piadina on both sides for about 3 minutes. Stuff as you like.

NUTRITION:

Calories 262 Carbs 24g Fat 15g Protein 8g

18) Mushroom velouté

INGREDIENTS:

- ➤ 1 cup thick coconut milk
- ➤ cups fresh mushrooms
- ➤ Salt
- ➤ Pepper
- ➤ Parsley
- ➤ Chili pepper (Optional)

DIRECTIONS:

1. Place the mushrooms in a large nonstick pot.
2. Add parsley, salt and pepper and 2 tablespoons of water.
3. Close with a lid and simmer for 10 minutes. Add coconut milk and continue cooking for 15-20 minutes.
4. Remove from heat, let cool slightly and blend (you can set aside a few mushrooms to garnish the dish).

NUTRITION:

Calories 100 Carbs 8g Fat 5g Protein 7g

19) Savory crêpe

INGREDIENTS:

- 3 eggs
- 3 tablespoons almond flour
- 2 tablespoons fresh soft cheese
- 2 tablespoons liquid cream
- Salt

DIRECTIONS:

1. In a small pan, melt the cheese with the cream over very low heat.
2. Put it in a bowl and add the eggs, flour and salt, then mix with the help of an electric mixer until you get a smooth mixture.
3. Let stand for a few moments and then proceed with the classic cooking process for crêpes.
4. Stuff as you prefer, for example with ricotta and spinach.

NUTRITION:

Calories 497 Carbs 12g Fat 38g Protein 27g

20) Savory plum cake

INGREDIENTS:

- 1 cup egg whites
- 5 ounces diced assorted cold cuts
- 1/4 cup grated mozzarella cheese
- 1/4 cup linseed flour
- 1/4 cup diced cheddar
- 1/4 cup grated Parmesan cheese
- 2 tablespoons pitted and chopped black olives
- 1 1/2 tablespoons extra virgin olive oil
- 1/2 sachet yeast
- Salt and pepper

DIRECTIONS:

1. In a bowl put all the ingredients.
2. Simply mix everything with an electric mixer and bake at 345° F (175° C) for about 35 minutes in a 9-inch plum cake pan, buttered and floured with bamboo fiber.

NUTRITION:

Calories 654 Carbs 12g Fat 38g Protein 66g

21) Quiche Lorraine
(French savory pie)

INGREDIENTS for an 8 x 2 inch round mold:

For the base:

- 4 sachets (1 cup) Tisanoreica gluten-free flour
- for bread
- 1/4 cup butter
- 1 egg
- 1 1/2 tablespoons grated Parmesan cheese, aged 24 months
- Salt and pepper
- 1 pinch baking powder

For the appareil (cream and egg mixture):
- 3/4 cup milk
- 3/4 cup water
- 3 eggs
- 1/2 cup bacon cubes
- 1/2 cup Gruyere cubes
- Salt and pepper

DIRECTIONS:

1. For the base, mix in a bowl the butter with the egg, Parmesan cheese, salt and pepper. Then add the Tisanoreica gluten-free flour and the yeast. Roll out the dough and line the mold.
2. Bake at 340° F (170° C) for 10 minutes.
3. Brown the bacon in a pan without adding anything else.
4. Put on the cooked base along with Gruyere cubes.
5. Prepare the appareil by mixing the milk, water and eggs.
6. Also add salt and pepper. Pour the appareil on the cooked base and complete cooking in the oven at 340° F (170° C) for at least 45 minutes (insert a toothpick in the center of the quiche, if it comes out dry the pie is ready).

NUTRITION:

Calories 1295 Carbs 21g Fat 99g Protein 81g

12
LUNCH RECIPES

1) Beef meatballs on zucchini and valerian pesto

INGREDIENTS:

For the meatballs:

- 3/4 cup lean ground beef
- Fresh herbs to taste
- Salt
- Pepper
- Garlic

For the pesto:

- 1/2 cup zucchini
- 1/4 cup valerian
- 1/4 cup water
- Chili pepper to taste

DIRECTIONS:

1. Shape the meatballs by mixing the meat with the herbs.
2. Cook for 5 minutes in an air fryer. In the meantime, prepare the pesto.
3. Wash and dry the zucchini, cut it into chunks and put it in a mixer with valerian, chili pepper, salt and water.
4. Pour the pesto on the plate and place the meatballs on it.

NUTRITION:

Calories 136 Carbs 8g Fat 4g Protein 16g

2) Bolivian style veal in basket

INGREDIENTS:

- 2 leaves romaine lettuce, washed and dried
- ounces veal strips
- 1/2 bell pepper
- 1 zucchini
- A little onion
- Spices (pepper, cumin, chili pepper, oregano)
- Salt

DIRECTIONS:

1. Sauté the onion, add the peppers and zucchini cut into strips and let cook for 10 minutes.
2. Add the meat and spices, let the flavors blend and salt to taste.
3. Put the two lettuce leaves on the bottom of a small basket and fill with the meat.

NUTRITION:

Calories 68 Carbs 12g Fat 2g Protein 4g

3) Braciole (stuffed Italian meat rolls)

INGREDIENTS:

- ➢ slices veal
- ➢ 1 cup pecorino cheese
- ➢ 1 garlic clove
- ➢ 1 sprig parsley
- ➢ Salt to taste
- ➢ Pepper to taste
- ➢ 1/2 cup white wine
- ➢ 2 cups tomato pulp
- ➢ 1/4 cup golden onion
- ➢ 1/2 cup extra virgin olive oil

DIRECTIONS:

1. Chop the garlic and parsley and grate the pecorino cheese.
2. Lay the meat slices on a flat surface and stuff with the prepared seasoning, a pinch of salt and pepper.
3. Roll up each slice to form a roll which you will then close with kitchen twine or toothpicks. Finely slice the onion and fry it with the oil in a fairly large pan.
4. Add the braciole and brown them evenly. Pour in the wine and cook until the alcohol has completely evaporated.
5. Add the tomato puree diluted with one or two glasses of water, add salt and cook for at least 1 hour with the lid on and over low heat.

NUTRITION:

Calories 438 Carbs 15g Fat 38g Protein 9g

4) Chicken breast en croute and fennel with lemon

INGREDIENTS for 1 serving:

- ➢ Chicken breast
- ➢ Fennel
- ➢ Butter, lemon and thyme
- ➢ For the croute:
- ➢ 3/4 cup almond flour
- ➢ 1/4 cup flaxseed flour
- ➢ 2 1/2 tablespoons psyllium
- ➢ 2 egg whites
- ➢ 1 tablespoon water
- ➢ Chives
- ➢ Oregano
- ➢ Salt

DIRECTIONS:

1. For the croute, mix the dry ingredients, then add the liquid ones.
2. Let the dough stand for 10 minutes. Spread it between 2 sheets of baking paper greased with olive oil.
3. Brush the dough with mustard seeds and lay the chicken breast.
4. Close first crosswise, then lengthwise like an envelope.
5. Bake at 340° F (170° C) for 50 minutes until golden brown. Sauté the fennel in butter, lemon and thyme and serve it with the chicken.

NUTRITION:

Calories 525 Carbs 27g Fat 23g Protein 53g

5) Chicken breast with paprika

INGREDIENTS:

- ➤ 2-3 whole chicken breasts
- ➤ 4 tablespoons sweet paprika
- ➤ Salt to taste
- ➤ Ground black pepper
- ➤ 2-3 tablespoons extra virgin olive oil
- ➤ Lemon
- ➤ Spices to taste

DIRECTIONS:

1. Divide the chicken breasts in half, lay them in a dish and sprinkle them with lemon, letting them stand for about 10 minutes. In a bowl, mix the sweet paprika with a pinch of ground black pepper.
2. Now drain the chicken breasts and pat them dry with paper towels, then sprinkle them with extra virgin olive oil and massage them all around.
3. Dip them in the paprika, pressing lightly on the meat so that the spice adheres on all sides.
4. At this point, place the chicken breast fillets between two sheets of baking paper and gently beat them with a meat tenderizer.
5. Take a griddle (a cast iron one if possible), heat it and place the chicken breasts on it.
6. Add a little oil. Cook over medium-high heat for about 3-4 minutes per side, so that the outside is crispy and the inside is soft and juicy.
7. Finally cut the chicken breast fillets into slanted slices and serve them with a vegetable side dish.

NUTRITION:

Calories 900 Carbs 5g Fat 54g Protein 98g

6) Chicken escalopes with saffron sauce

INGREDIENTS:

- ➤ ounces chicken escalopes
- ➤ Bamboo fiber to bread to taste
- ➤ Black salt
- ➤ Pepper
- ➤ 1/4 cup thick coconut milk
- ➤ 1 sachet saffron
- ➤ 1 dab clarified butter

DIRECTIONS:

1. Season the chicken escalopes with salt and pepper and lightly flour them.
2. Cook them in a pan with butter. When cooked, transfer to a serving dish.
3. In the pot, let the coconut milk thicken with saffron and garnish the escalopes.

NUTRITION:

Calories 365 Carbs 1g Fat 19g Protein 48g

7) Chicken strips with arugula pesto

INGREDIENTS:

- ➤ For the arugula pesto:
- ➤ 4 cups arugula
- ➤ 1/2 cup walnuts
- ➤ 1 garlic clove
- ➤ 1/2 cup Parmesan cheese
- ➤ 1 pinch salt
- ➤ 3/4 cup extra virgin olive oil
- ➤ For the chicken strips:
- ➤ 1 pound chicken breast
- ➤ Extra virgin olive oil to taste
- ➤ Salt and pepper to taste
- ➤ Grated Parmesan cheese to taste

DIRECTIONS:

1. Put all the ingredients for the pesto in a blender and blend at full speed.
2. Cut the chicken breast into strips. In a bowl, moisten the chicken with plenty of extra virgin olive oil and dip it in grated Parmesan cheese.
3. Place in a baking sheet lined with baking paper, add salt, pepper and more grated Parmesan cheese and bake at 390° F (200° C) until golden brown.
4. Serve with the arugula pesto.

NUTRITION:

Calories 1598 Carbs 22g Fat 121g Protein 104g

8) Chicken strips with coconut

INGREDIENTS:

- ➤ 1 cup chicken strips
- ➤ 1/4 cup coconut flour
- ➤ 2 eggs
- ➤ 1/2 cup shredded coconut
- ➤ Salt and pepper

DIRECTIONS:

1. Mix coconut flour with salt and pepper. Flour the strips and dip them in the egg.
2. Bread them in the shredded coconut and arrange them on a baking sheet.
3. Grease everything with a little extra virgin olive oil.

4. Bake at 390° F (200° C) for 25 minutes, turning them halfway through cooking.

NUTRITION:

Calories 647 Carbs 18g Fat 33g Protein 68g

9) Chicken with capers and lemon

INGREDIENTS:

- ➤ ounces boneless chicken thighs (without skin)
- ➤ salt
- ➤ pepper
- ➤ 1 tablespoon coconut oil
- ➤ 1 teaspoon lemon juice
- ➤ 1/4 cup capers

DIRECTIONS:

1. Dry the chicken thighs with paper towel. Add salt and pepper on both sides.
2. Cook in the coconut oil over medium heat.
3. Add capers and lemon juice and cook for 15-20 minutes with a lid on.

NUTRITION:

Calories 464 Carbs 1g Fat 34g Protein 38g

10) Chicken with cream of coconut milk and curry, zucchini, Tropea onion and "snow" of toasted almonds

INGREDIENTS for 2 people:

- 14 ounces chicken strips
- 3/4 cup thick coconut milk
- 2 tablespoons coconut oil
- 2 tablespoons coconut flour
- 1 cup zucchini
- 1/2 cup Tropea onion
- 1 dash white wine
- 1/4 cup chopped almonds
- Curry mix (sweet, hot and Bombay)
- 1 tablespoon soy sauce

DIRECTIONS:

1. Dice zucchini and onion. In a pan, heat coconut oil for 1 minute and sauté zucchini and onion together for about 5 minutes over high heat.
2. In the meantime, put the coconut flour in a dish with the spices, stir and flour the strips.
3. Add the strips to the pan and fry on all sides over high heat for about 5 minutes. Simmer with wine and add the coconut milk and soy sauce, lower the heat and continue to cook until the sauce has thickened.
4. Add most of the almonds and use the remaining to decorate the dish.

NUTRITION:

Calories 956 Carbs 22g Fat 30g Protein 98g

11) Chicken with mushrooms

INGREDIENTS:

- 1 cup field mushrooms
- 1 chicken breast cut into thick slices
- Coconut flour
- Extra virgin olive oil
- Garlic powder
- Salt and pepper

DIRECTIONS:

1. Grease a pan with extra virgin olive oil. Flour the chicken breast slices.
2. Place the meat in the pan and turn it when browned. Repeat on the other side. Top with sliced mushrooms.
3. Add garlic and season with salt and pepper.
4. Cover with water and simmer to obtain desired creaminess.

NUTRITION:

Calories 556 Carbs 20g Fat 36g Protein 39g

12) Chicken with turmeric

INGREDIENTS:

- 4 ounces chicken breast cut into very thin slices
- 3/4 cup onion cut into thin slices
- Turmeric to taste
- Coconut flour to taste
- 1 tablespoon extra virgin olive oil
- Salt and pepper

DIRECTIONS:

1. Heat the extra virgin olive oil in a nonstick pan and brown the onions.
2. Lightly flour the chicken breast and brown it in the pan along with the onions.
3. Add turmeric, salt and pepper to taste.
4. Pour in a little water and allow to evaporate over low heat.

NUTRITION:

Calories 450 Carbs 24g Fat 24g Protein 34g

13) Crispy chicken fillets with cheese

INGREDIENTS for 1 serving:

- 1 1/2 tablespoons Lo Dough breadcrumbs
- 1 1/2 tablespoons shredded Groksi (crispy pieces of dried cheese) or grated Parmesan cheese
- 1 boneless chicken breast cut into fillets
- 1 small egg, beaten
- Cooking oil spray

DIRECTIONS:

1. Preheat the oven to 430° F (220° C). Put the beaten egg in a bowl and the breadcrumbs mixed with the Groksi in another.
2. Dip the chicken fillets first in the egg and then in the breadcrumbs, shaking them to remove excess breadcrumbs (if you want an even crisper and thicker crust, repeat the process twice).
3. Place the breaded fillets on a baking sheet lined with baking paper, drizzle with oil and bake for 20 minutes, turning at around 3/4 of the time (the cooking time varies depending on the size of the chicken fillets).

NUTRITION:

Calories 449 Carbs 9g Fat 26g Protein 46g

14) Eggs "in purgatory" (with tomato sauce)

INGREDIENTS:

- 3 eggs
- Salt
- Pepper
- 1 garlic clove
- Oil
- Grated Parmesan cheese to taste
- Fresh basil
- 1 cup tomato sauce

DIRECTIONS:

1. In a nonstick pan, brown the garlic with a drizzle of oil.
2. Remove the garlic, add the tomato sauce.

Stir and create "holes" where you will gently insert the eggs.
3. Season with salt and pepper and close with a lid. Cook for 5/7 minutes
4. Sprinkle with Parmesan cheese and add fresh basil.

NUTRITION:

Calories 235 Carbs 2g Fat 16g Protein 21g

15) Gnocchi with butter, sage and lemon

INGREDIENTS for 2 servings:

- 2 cups almond flour
- 1 tablespoon psyllium husk
- 1 tablespoon xanthan gum
- 1 egg
- 1 tablespoon extra virgin olive oil
- 1 tablespoon water
- 1 pinch salt
- Butter
- Sage leaves
- Lemon peel

DIRECTIONS:

1. Blend all the ingredients for a few seconds, so that everything is well mixed.
2. Knead with your hands and shape long and thin rolls. Cut out small chunks and shape them into gnocchi.
3. Mark them with the prongs of a fork. Fry for a few minutes with plenty of butter, some sage leaves and lemon peel.

NUTRITION:

Calories 1493 Carbs 58g Fat 116g Protein 54g

16) Goulash (Hungarian meat soup)

INGREDIENTS:

- ➢ ounces beef bites
- ➢ 2 cups onion
- ➢ Extra virgin olive oil
- ➢ Sweet paprika
- ➢ Salt and pepper

DIRECTIONS:

1. In a pan, heat 2 tablespoons of extra virgin olive oil.
2. Chop the onion into large pieces and brown it with the meat. Put everything in the pressure cooker, add salt and pepper to taste.
3. You can also add bay leaves and a little cumin. Pour in some water and cook for 20 minutes.
4. Remove the lid and add the sweet paprika. Continue to cook over low heat.

NUTRITION:

Calories 536 Carbs 30g Fat280g Protein 41g

17) Ground meat triangles

INGREDIENTS:

- ➢ 3 ounces ground meat mix
- ➢ 1 slice processed cheese
- ➢ 1 slice ham

DIRECTIONS:

1. Roll out the ground meat forming a square. Cut out 4 triangles.
2. Take a triangle and top it with 1/2 slice of processed cheese and 1/2 slice of ham, then close it with another triangle.
3. Repeat to make another one. Cook in a pan for 3 minutes per side.

NUTRITION:

Calories 203 Carbs 4g Fat 11g Protein 22g

18) Keto cacio e pepe (pasta with black pepper and pecorino cheese)

Ingredients for 2 people:

- ➢ 1 1/2 cup gluten-free rotini pasta by Tisanoreica
- ➢ 1 cup grated PDO pecorino romano cheese
- ➢ High quality black pepper grains

DIRECTIONS:

1. Boil some water with a little salt, pour in the pasta and cook for 15-18 minutes.
2. Put the pecorino romano cheese in a bowl and make a cream by pouring a little cooking water of the pasta.
3. Let the pasta stand in water off the heat for 3 minutes.
4. Crush the pepper and toast it in a pan, pour in the pasta and sauté.
5. Remove from heat and mix with the pecorino romano cream.
6. If you like, you can add some truffle flakes or grated bottarga (a delicacy of salted, cured fish roe).

NUTRITION:

Calories 848 Carbs 108g Fat 28g Protein 40g

19) Keto cannelloni (cylindrical type of lasagna) with shrimps and black cabbage

INGREDIENTS:

- ➢ 1 egg
- ➢ 1/4 cup cream cheese
- ➢ 2 leaves black cabbage
- ➢ 2 ounces shrimps
- ➢ 1/4 cup crescenza cheese
- ➢ Olive oil
- ➢ Salt
- ➢ Garlic
- ➢ Keto white sauce
- ➢ Parmesan cheese

DIRECTIONS:

1. First prepare the puff pastry for the cannelloni by mixing the egg with the cream cheese. Spread on a 7 x 7-in square nonstick pan.
2. While the puff pastry is cooling, sauté in a pan the black cabbage cut into strips with oil, garlic and chili pepper for a few minutes. In the same pan, blanch the shrimps.
3. Once the pastry has cooled, divide it in half to make two cannelloni.
4. Spread the crescenza cheese on the puff pastry and add the black cabbage and shrimps.
5. Roll up carefully and place in a baking sheet. Sprinkle the cannelloni with plenty of white sauce and Parmesan cheese. Bake at 390° F (200° C) for 15 minutes or until golden brown.

NUTRITION:

Calories 713 Carbs 9g Fat 63g Protein 27g

20) Keto lasagna

INGREDIENTS:

For the dough:

- ➢ 1 1/2 cups RevoMix Pasta flour by Revolution03
- ➢ 2 medium-sized eggs
- ➢ 1/4 cup water
- ➢ For the white sauce:
- ➢ 1/2 cup lactose-free cream
- ➢ 1/4 cup ghee
- ➢ 1/2 cup lactose-free Philadelphia
- ➢ Salt
- ➢ Nutmeg
- ➢ 1 teaspoon xanthan

DIRECTIONS:

1. Mix all the ingredient for the dough in the kneader and let it stand for 60 minutes in the fridge.
2. With a dough sheeter, roll out the dough. Cut it into discs and set aside.
3. In a small pan heat the milk with the butter, salt and nutmeg.
4. As soon as the mixture is hot, add the Philadelphia and stir vigorously. Let it boil, remove from heat and add the xanthan.
5. Prepare the dish as a normal lasagna by using the dough discs, the white sauce and meat sauce (slow cooked for 6 hours).

NUTRITION:

Calories 884 Carbs 59g Fat 59g Protein 29g

21) Keto ravioli (stuffed pasta similar to dumplings)

INGREDIENTS:

- 3/4 cups flour for pasta by Revolution03
- 1 medium-sized egg
- 1 tablespoon water

DIRECTIONS:

1. Beat the egg with the water and add to the flour on a pastry board. Knead with your hands until you get a smooth and homogeneous dough.
2. Wrap with plastic wrap and let stand in the fridge for about an hour.
3. Roll out the dough, possibly with the appropriate tool or with a rolling pin. Stuff as you like (for example with fish filling).
4. Shape the ravioli and cook for 8/9 minutes. Check the cooking time as you like. Season to taste.

NUTRITION:

Calories 528 Carbs 82g Fat 10g Protein 27g

22) Keto shepherd's pie

INGREDIENTS for 2 generous servings:

- 14 ounces ground beef or lamb
- 3 cups cauliflower
- 1/4 cup cooking cream
- 1 egg
- 1/4 cup yellow butter or grass-fed butter
- 1/4 cup grated Parmesan cheese
- 1 tablespoon mayonnaise (optional)
- Salt and pepper to taste

DIRECTIONS:

1. Preheat the oven to 390° F (200° C). Steam the cauliflower until well cooked and blend it to obtain a puree.
2. Then add the cream, Parmesan cheese, egg, salt and pepper and mix everything together.
3. Separately, cook the ground meat in butter and add the mayonnaise, salt and pepper or your favorite spices.

4. Put the meat in a baking sheet and cover it with the cauliflower puree. Bake for about 20-25 minutes.

NUTRITION:

Calories 1076 Carbs 19g Fat 65g Protein 103g

23) Konjac rice with mushrooms

INGREDIENTS:

- 1/4 cup konjac rice
- 2 tablespoons milk
- 1/4 cup onion
- 1 tablespoon Parmesan cheese
- 1 tablespoon extra virgin olive oil
- Vegetable broth to taste
- Mushrooms

DIRECTIONS:

1. Lightly sauté the onion and put the rice into the pan, toast it for a few minutes and then add a little broth.
2. In the meantime, soak the mushrooms in milk, then add them to the rice.
3. After 15 minutes, the rice will be cooked. Sprinkle with Parmesan cheese and add a drizzle of balsamic vinegar and a pinch of sage.

NUTRITION:

Calories 241 Carbs 13g Fat 17g Protein 10g

24) Mushrooms au gratin

INGREDIENTS:

- Mushrooms
- 2 tablespoons almond flour
- 2 tablespoons flaxseed flour
- Garlic
- Parsley
- Salt
- Extra virgin olive oil
- 1/2 cup water

DIRECTIONS:

1. Chop the garlic and mix all the ingredients. Use this mixture to bread the mushrooms.
2. Bake in the oven at 355° F (180° C) for about 40 minutes.

NUTRITION:

Calories 171 Carbs 10g Fat 10g Protein 10g

25) Mushroom stuffed with pistachio

INGREDIENTS:

- 1 large mushroom (about 14 ounces)
- 1/4 cup cream
- 1/4 cup pistachio pesto
- 1/4 cup stretched-curd cheese
- Parmesan cheese
- Chopped pistachios
- Pistachio flour

DIRECTIONS:

1. Remove the stem of the mushroom and hollow out the inside slightly.
2. Wash, dry and pierce the inside with a fork.
3. Line a baking sheet with baking paper. Mix cream and pesto.
4. Fill the mushroom with cheese, cream and pesto mixture, Parmesan cheese and chopped pistachios.
5. Cover with foil and finally bake at 390° F (200° C) for 20 minutes.
6. Remove the foil and continue baking for 3 minutes in grill mode, maximum power.
7. Put in the plate and finish with a sprinkle of pistachio flour.

NUTRITION:

Calories 434 Carbs 10g Fat 32g Protein 26g

26) Noodle omelet

INGREDIENTS:

- nests Shirataki noodles
- 1 tablespoon clarified butter
- 2 eggs
- 1/4 cup Parmesan cheese
- 1/4 cup bacon
- 1/2 cup assorted cheeses (whatever you have in the fridge!)
- Olive oil
- Salt and pepper to taste

DIRECTIONS:

1. Cook noodles according to package directions. Once salted and cooked, drain and add butter, then let cool.
2. Beat eggs with salt, pepper, Parmesan cheese, add bacon and cheeses and mix with the noodles.
3. Prepare a pan with a drizzle of oil and heat it, add the noodles and cook over low heat. After about 5 minutes, a golden crust will form. Turn with the help of a plate or lid, another 5 minutes and it's ready! You can eat hot or cold.

NUTRITION:

Calories 604 Carbs 11g Fat 52g Protein 22g

27) Oriental style noodles

INGREDIENTS for 2 servings:

- ➢ 1 bell pepper
- ➢ 1 small carrot
- ➢ 1/2 onion
- ➢ 2 savoy cabbage leaves
- ➢ 3 cups shiitake mushrooms
- ➢ 3 cups shirataki noodles
- ➢ 3 tablespoons coconut oil

DIRECTIONS:

1. Sauté the carrot with 1 tablespoon of coconut oil, then remove it from the pot.
2. Sauté the pepper with another tablespoon of coconut oil, then remove it from the pot.
3. Lower the heat and sauté the onion with another tablespoon of coconut oil, together with the mushrooms and cabbage.
4. Cook with the lid on for a few minutes adding the soy sauce (season with little salt because the soy sauce is already salty).
5. When the vegetables have softened, remove them and set aside.
6. In the hot pot, sauté the shirataki noodles, previously washed under cold water, to remove all excess water.
7. Add all the vegetables and mix. Serve hot and eat with chopsticks.

NUTRITION:

Calories 660 Carbs 54g Fat 43g Protein 15g

28) Pseudo carbonara

with zucchini and bacon

INGREDIENTS:

- ➢ Tagliatelle pasta by Le Gamberi Ketogenic Foods
- ➢ 1 large zucchini
- ➢ A few slices bacon
- ➢ 1 egg
- ➢ Bamboo flour
- ➢ Grated pecorino cheese
- ➢ Spices

DIRECTIONS:

1. Cut the zucchini into strips and dip them in beaten egg with spices to taste, then bread with a mixture of bamboo flour, pecorino, pepper and garlic powder.
2. Bake them in the air fryer for 12 minutes at 355° F (180° C).
3. At 5 minutes, put the bacon and raise to 375° F (190° C).
4. In the meantime, cook the pasta and then mix it with the remaining beaten egg. Add the zucchini and crispy bacon.

NUTRITION:

Calories 476 Carbs 24g Fat 15g Protein 24g

29) Pulled pork

INGREDIENTS for 2 people:

- ➢ 14 ounces pork loin
- ➢ Salt
- ➢ Pepper
- ➢ 6-7 fresh strawberries, cleaned and sliced
- ➢ Fresh basil leaves
- ➢ 1 teaspoon coconut or apple vinegar
- ➢ Olive oil
- ➢ 4-5 slices salami, cut into thin strips

DIRECTIONS:

1. Generously season the pork on both sides with salt and pepper and let stand at room temperature for about 20 minutes.
2. In the meantime, put the strawberries, basil, vinegar, olive oil and a pinch of salt and pepper in a bowl.
3. Stir and set aside for 15 minutes. Preheat the oven to 390° F (200° C).
4. Heat the oil in a large pan, add the pork and brown on both sides until golden brown (about 3 minutes per side).
5. Transfer to a baking sheet and bake for 10-15 minutes or until cooked through.
6. While the pork is cooking, season the salami with the strawberries and basil. Cut the pork and serve with the basil and strawberry mixture.

NUTRITION:

Calories 640 Carbs 7g Fat 32g Protein 81g

30) Red rice pie with lentils and zucchini

INGREDIENTS for 1 person:

- 1/2 cup whole red rice
- 1/4 cup peeled red lentils
- 2 zucchinis
- 1 tablespoon olive oil

DIRECTIONS:

1. Cook the rice in boiling salted water for 35 minutes.
2. Meanwhile, cook the lentils for 15 minutes. Once cooked, blend with a tablespoon of oil. Cut the zucchinis into cubes and cook them in a nonstick pan.
3. Combine the rice, lentils and zucchini and arrange in a ring mold. Let cool before removing it.

NUTRITION:

Calories 639 Carbs 105g Fat 15g Protein 21g

31) Stewed tripe

INGREDIENTS:

- 2 pounds tripe
- 1 golden onion
- 3 celery stalks
- 2 garlic cloves
- Salt to taste
- Olive oil to taste
- Wine to taste
- Capers to taste
- 1 hot chili pepper
- 2 1/2 cups peeled tomatoes
- Grated Parmesan cheese to taste

DIRECTIONS:

1. Cut the tripe into not too thin strips, rinse several times in fresh water and drain in a colander.
2. In a pan, pour plenty of extra virgin olive oil and the chopped celery, onion and garlic. Sauté over low heat for 5 minutes.
3. At this point, add the tripe and salt to the mixture, let gain flavor and pour in the wine.
4. Once the alcohol has evaporated, add the peeled tomatoes, capers and chili pepper.
5. Cover and cook over low heat for about 2 hours, turning from time to time. If necessary, add a little hot water.
6. The tripe is ready when it has become tender, but still retains its characteristic callosity. With the heat off, add plenty of grated Parmesan cheese. Let gain flavor for a few minutes and serve while still hot.

NUTRITION:

Calories 528 Carbs 29g Fat 26g Protein 45g

32) Stringy meatloaf with black cabbage chips

INGREDIENTS:

- ➢ 3 cups black cabbage
- ➢ ounces minced veal
- ➢ ounces sausage
- ➢ 1 egg
- ➢ 3/4 cup cheese (such as Asiago) to taste
- ➢ 4 ounces cooked ham
- ➢ 4 tablespoons Parmesan cheese
- ➢ Herbs
- ➢ Salt and pepper

DIRECTIONS:

1. Wash the black cabbage leaves and remove the middle, tough part. Then mix the two meats with the herbs (such as semi-fresh basil), salt and pepper, egg and Parmesan cheese.
2. Let stand in the fridge while you prepare the black cabbage.
3. With your hands, break some of the leaves into squares of about 1 inch per side.
4. Cut the remaining leaves into thin strips and fry them with a little olive oil and a garlic clove. Season the leaves for the chips with oil, salt and yacón.
5. Put them on a baking sheet lined with baking paper without overlapping and bake in the fan oven for 15 minutes at 300° F (150° C) being careful not to let them burn.
6. Then take the meats and lay them on the baking paper.
7. Fill with the cooked ham, sautéed black cabbage and cheese. Roll up and let stand in the fridge for 1 hour. Season with extra virgin olive oil and bake in the fan oven at 375° F (190° C) for 35/40 minutes.

NUTRITION:

Calories 655 Carbs 19g Fat 42g Protein 50g

33) Stuffed meat pie

INGREDIENTS:

- ➢ For the base:
- ➢ 1 pound minced meat
- ➢ 1/2 cup fresh cream
- ➢ 2/3 cup Parmesan cheese
- ➢ 1 whole egg
- ➢ Salt
- ➢ Parsley
- ➢ Basil
- ➢ Garlic
- ➢ Pepper
- ➢ For the filling:
- ➢ Mushrooms
- ➢ Mozzarella cheese for pizza

DIRECTIONS:

1. Prepare the base for the pie by mixing all the ingredients listed, as if making a meatloaf.
2. If it is too liquid, put more Parmesan cheese. If it is too thick, put more cream. In an 8-inch mold, put half of the meat mixture.
3. Cook the mushrooms in olive oil, parsley and garlic. Cover the base with the mushrooms and mozzarella and close with the other half of the meat mixture.
4. Sprinkle the pie with mozzarella and Parmesan cheese and bake at 390° F (200° C) for 25/30 minutes.

NUTRITION:

Calories 1109 Carbs 4g Fat 73g Protein 109g

34) Stuffed mushrooms

INGREDIENTS:

- ➤ Mushrooms
- ➤ 3 ounces fresh spinach
- ➤ ounces minced meat
- ➤ 2 slices keto bread
- ➤ 1 egg
- ➤ 1/3 cup almond milk
- ➤ 2 tablespoons Parmesan cheese
- ➤ 2 tablespoons grated gouda cheese
- ➤ Fresh parsley
- ➤ Fresh spring onion
- ➤ Fresh oregano
- ➤ 1 garlic clove, crushed
- ➤ Pepper and salt to taste
- ➤ 2 tablespoons extra virgin olive oil

DIRECTIONS:

1. Clean the mushrooms with a cloth, remove the stems and brush with oil and salt inside and out.
2. In a bowl, mix the meat with the other ingredients, including the stems of the chopped mushrooms, and then use this mixture to stuff the mushrooms.
3. Bake at 430° F (220° C) for 25 minutes.

NUTRITION:

Calories 824 Carbs 7g Fat 69g Protein 43g

35) Tuna and ricotta cheese meatballs

INGREDIENTS for 3/4 people:

- ➤ 1 cup grated Parmesan cheese
- ➤ 2 eggs
- ➤ 2 sprigs parsley, finely chopped
- ➤ 1 cup drained tuna in olive oil
- ➤ 1/2 cup drained fresh ricotta cheese
- ➤ 1/2 teaspoon salt
- ➤ Oil for frying
- ➤ Almond flour to bread the meatballs

DIRECTIONS:

1. Mix the Parmesan cheese, parsley, tuna, ricotta, 1 egg, salt, pepper and almond flour If needed to make the mixture more compact. Place the mixture in the fridge for an hour to let it thicken, it will then be easier to shape the balls. In a bowl beat the remaining egg, and in another one put the almond flour.
2. With slightly wet hands, shape the meatballs and then dip them first in the egg and then in the flour.
3. Fry them in a pan with seed oil, then lay them on a plate with paper towel to dry the excess oil.

NUTRITION:

Calories 909 Carbs 16g Fat 57g Protein 83g

36) Turkey chunks with curry-flavored coconut milk

INGREDIENTS:

- ➤ 1 pound turkey chunks
- ➤ 1 cup coconut milk
- ➤ 1 tablespoon curry powder
- ➤ 1 teaspoon ginger
- ➤ Lemon peel
- ➤ 1/4 teaspoon xanthan
- ➤ Salt, chili pepper and thyme
- ➤ Extra virgin olive oil

DIRECTIONS:

1. In a large pan, brown the turkey with extra virgin olive oil, thyme and chili pepper.
2. In a small pan, heat the coconut milk with curry powder, ginger, lemon peel and salt.
3. When the turkey is browned, add the coconut sauce and cook for 40 minutes over low heat.
4. Stir occasionally. 10 minutes before turning off, add the xanthan. Serve warm.

NUTRITION:

Calories 694 Carbs 20g Fat 23g Protein 102g

13

SEAFOOD & FISH RECIPES

1) Asian style salmon

INGREDIENTS:

- ➢ 3 cups frozen vegetables
- ➢ ounces salmon fillet
- ➢ Salt and chili flakes
- ➢ 2 tablespoons lemon juice
- ➢ 2 tablespoons soy sauce
- ➢ 1 teaspoon tahini sauce
- ➢ 1 teaspoon sesame seeds

DIRECTIONS:

1. Arrange the frozen vegetables on the bottom of the slow cooker.
2. Sprinkle the salmon with salt and pepper. Arrange it on top of the vegetables.
3. Stir in the lemon juice, soy and tahini. Pour the mixture over the salmon and sprinkle with sesame seeds. Cook over low heat for 3 hours.

NUTRITION:

Calories 672 Carbs 74g Fat 21g Protein 47g

2) Codfish au gratin

INGREDIENTS for 2 people:

- ➢ 5 ounces cod
- ➢ 1 serving Pnk rusks
- ➢ Iodized salt to taste
- ➢ Lemon thyme
- ➢ Extra virgin olive oil
- ➢ Peppers and potatoes to taste

DIRECTIONS:

1. Finely chop the rusks and lemon thyme.
2. Grease the cod and bread it in the breadcrumbs obtained from the rusks.
3. Cook in the pan along with the vegetables for 2 minutes per side.

NUTRITION:

Calories 310 Carbs 14g Fat 17g Protein 25g

3) Codfish meatballs in Parmesan cheese basket with red radicchio and walnut salad

INGREDIENTS:

- For 13 meatballs:
- 5 ounces codfish, drained and chopped
- 1 tablespoon psyllium
- 1/4 cup egg whites
- Spices (such as fennel seeds)
- For the basket:
- 2 tablespoons Parmesan cheese
- For the salad:
- 4 ounces long red radicchio
- 2 radishes
- 1 chopped walnut
- Salt, oil and apple cider vinegar

DIRECTIONS:

1. Form the meatballs by mixing the listed ingredients.
2. For the basket, put the Parmesan cheese in a 4-5 inch pan, let it melt and thicken.
3. Take it with a spatula and put it in a bowl upside down.
4. Be quick because it hardens quickly.
5. Serve the meatballs in the Parmesan cheese basket and add the salad prepared by mixing the listed ingredients.

NUTRITION:

Calories 299 Carbs 14g Fat 10g Protein 38g

4) Fried salmon with pumpkin and sesame seeds

INGREDIENTS:

- 1 salmon slice
- 2 tablespoons butter
- Sesame seeds
- Chopped pumpkin seeds
- Salt and pepper

DIRECTIONS:

1. Melt the butter in a small pan.
2. Dice the salmon and fry it in the butter.
3. Add the chopped sesame and pumpkin seeds when the salmon is almost cooked and toast them.

NUTRITION:

Calories 268 Carbs 3g Fat 24g Protein 10g

5) Green omelet roll with salmon

INGREDIENTS:

- 5 cups arugula
- Pine nuts
- 1/4 cup Parmesan cheese
- 6 eggs
- Cream cheese
- ounces salmon
- Oil
- Salt
- Pepper

DIRECTIONS:

1. Blend the arugula, pine nuts, Parmesan cheese, salt, pepper and oil.
2. Add the eggs and blend again. Bake in the oven at 375° F (190° C) for 10 minutes.
3. Let cool, spread the cheese and then the salmon. Roll up and let stand in the fridge for at least 1 hour.

NUTRITION:

Calories 789 Carbs 18g Fat 47g Protein 74g

6) Grilled mackerel on leek fondue

INGREDIENTS:

- ➤ 1 grilled mackerel fillet
- ➤ 1 cup thinly sliced leeks
- ➤ Olive oil
- ➤ 1/2 tablespoon lemon juice
- ➤ 1/2 tablespoon mustard
- ➤ 1 tablespoon cream
- ➤ Salt and pepper

DIRECTIONS:

1. Fry the leeks in oil, let cook with the lid over low heat for a few minutes until soft.
2. Add the lemon juice, mustard, cream, salt and pepper.
3. Stir and allow to gain flavor for a few minutes. Arrange the grilled mackerel fillet on the fondue and drizzle with lemon oil.

NUTRITION:

Calories 479 Carbs 15g Fat 37g Protein 21g

7) Hawaiian style shrimps

INGREDIENTS:

- ➤ 2 medium-sized zucchinis
- ➤ 8-10 ounces frozen shrimps
- ➤ Coconut milk by Live Better
- ➤ Oil
- ➤ Garlic
- ➤ Curry
- ➤ Salt

DIRECTIONS:

1. Put oil in a pan and add the finely chopped garlic or garlic powder.
2. Add the zucchinis cut into squares or rounds and cook.
3. When more than halfway through cooking, add the shelled shrimps and after a couple of minutes add 3 cups of water, the curry and 4 scoops of coconut milk powder or just 1 cup of water and 2 cups of coconut milk. Salt to taste and allow the liquid to evaporate.

NUTRITION:

Calories 345 Carbs 13g Fat 7g Protein 58g

8) Keto teriyaki salmon with broccoli and mushrooms

INGREDIENTS:

- ➤ ounces salmon
- ➤ 1/2 onion, diced
- ➤ 3 1/2 cups broccoli
- ➤ 1 cup mushrooms
- ➤ 1/4 cup coconut aminos/soy sauce
- ➤ 2 tablespoons erythritol
- ➤ 1 garlic clove, chopped
- ➤ 1 teaspoon grated ginger

DIRECTIONS:

1. For the teriyaki sauce, mix coconut aminos (or soy sauce), erythritol, garlic and ginger in a small bowl.
2. Brush the salmon with some of the teriyaki sauce. Bake in the air fryer at 390° F (200° C) for 15 minutes.
3. Meanwhile, prepare the vegetable side dish by cooking the onion, broccoli and mushrooms in a pan over medium heat. Sauté for 5 minutes.
4. Pour in the remaining teriyaki sauce and continue to cook stirring occasionally, until the broccoli is tender. Serve and enjoy your teriyaki salmon with the vegetables.

NUTRITION:

Calories 324 Carbs 47g Fat 4g Protein 24g

9) Marinated salmon bites

INGREDIENTS:

- 2 salmon fillets
- 1/2 cup soy sauce
- 1 tablespoon tahini
- 1 small zucchini

DIRECTIONS:

1. First, mix soy sauce with tahini in a bowl, cut salmon into cubes and marinate for a few hours.
2. Cut the zucchini into thin slices with a peeler, wrap each salmon cube with a slice and close with a toothpick.
3. Bake in the oven at 355° F (180° C) for 20 minutes and serve with some sauce.
4. You can eat them with a simple Greek yogurt sauce seasoned with parsley, oil, a pinch of salt and a teaspoon of lemon juice.

NUTRITION:

Calories 597 Carbs 11g Fat 34g Protein 63g

10) Oriental style fish soup

INGREDIENTS:

- 1 pound mixed fish (for example 2 squids, 7 ounces pink shrimps, 2 scampi)
- 1 generous tablespoon coconut oil
- 3 cups broccoli
- 1 small onion
- 1 tablespoon garlic paste
- Juice of 1 lime
- 1 cup shellfish bisque*
- 2 tablespoons turmeric powder
- 1 teaspoon ginger powder
- Chili pepper
- 2/3 cup coconut milk
- Salt

DIRECTIONS:

1. Let the fish marinate for half an hour with the lime juice and turmeric.
2. Fry the thinly sliced onion and garlic paste in the coconut oil.
3. Add the raw broccoli cut into small pieces and cook for 5 minutes.

4. Add the remaining spices and salt, the bisque and coconut milk, and finally the fish. Let cook for about 10 minutes.
5. *Prepare the shellfish bisque by frying a small onion and 4 ripe Piccadilly tomatoes in olive oil, add a bunch of chopped parsley, the heads and shells of the crustaceans and crush to extract the juice. Pour in 1 cup of dry white wine and finally add 1 cup of water. Let cook for about 20 minutes over medium heat.

NUTRITION:

Calories 721 Carbs 33g Fat 21g Protein 99g

11) Salmon and avocado with oil in jar

INGREDIENTS for 2 people:

- ounces fresh salmon
- 1 avocado
- 4 cherry tomatoes
- Extra virgin olive oil to taste
- Organic lemon peel
- Garlic, thyme and fennel
- Salt and pepper

DIRECTIONS:

1. Remove the skin from the salmon and cut it into 1 inch cubes.
2. Season with a little olive oil, grated lemon peel, garlic, chopped herbs, salt and pepper. In the meantime, dice the avocado and remove the seeds from the cherry tomatoes, cutting them into small pieces.
3. Combine the seasoned salmon with the diced avocado and cherry tomatoes, mix carefully and place in two airtight jars.
4. Fill the jars with olive oil and seal them tightly.
5. Cook in a bain-marie over low heat for about 1 hour and a half.
6. This type of cooking is also perfect with shrimps and prawns.

NUTRITION:

Calories 468 Carbs 5g Fat 45g Protein 11g

12) Salmon burger

INGREDIENTS:

- ➢ 4 cans (about 10 ounces) salmon in olive oil
- ➢ 2 chopped spring onions (optional)
- ➢ 1/2 diced red bell pepper
- ➢ 2 tablespoons dill (or parsley)
- ➢ 1/4 cup almond flour
- ➢ 2 eggs
- ➢ 1 pinch sea salt
- ➢ 4 tablespoons extra virgin olive oil

DIRECTIONS:

1. Mix all the ingredients in a bowl, shred the salmon fillets and knead until smooth.
2. With your hands shape 4 balls which you will turn into burgers using a ring mold.
3. Heat a nonstick pan and place the burgers in it. Cook them for 3/4 minutes per side. Serve them with salad.

NUTRITION:

Calories 1477 Carbs 15g Fat 125g Protein 73g

13) Salmon en croute

INGREDIENTS:

- ➢ 2 fillets salmon
- ➢ 2 generous tablespoons hazelnut flour
- ➢ Parsley
- ➢ Pink pepper grains
- ➢ Lemon-flavored pepper
- ➢ Ginger
- ➢ Poppy seeds

DIRECTIONS:

1. In a small bowl, prepare the breadcrumbs by mixing the flavorings and hazelnut flour. Clean the fillets by removing any bones with the help of kitchen tongs.
2. Transfer the fillets into a baking sheet lined with baking paper and cover them with the breadcrumbs.
3. Bake in the preheated fan oven at 375° F (190° C) for about 20 minutes.

NUTRITION:

Calories 567 Carbs 3g Fat 36g Protein 58g

14) Salmon with pumpkin cream

INGREDIENTS for 1 person:

- ➢ 1/2 cup pumpkin
- ➢ 1 tablespoon Philadelphia cheese
- ➢ 4 ounces salmon fillet
- ➢ Salt, oil, pepper
- ➢ Chopped pistachios

DIRECTIONS:

1. Dice the pumpkin and set aside some smaller cubes.
2. Boil the pumpkin cubes and then blend them with the Philadelphia, oil, salt and pepper.
3. In the meantime, cook the salmon and the pumpkin cubes in the air fryer (you can also bake them in the oven).
4. Once the salmon is cooked, place it on the pumpkin cream and garnish with pumpkin cubes, chopped pistachios and a drizzle of oil.

NUTRITION:

Calories 226 Carbs 9g Fat 9g Protein 28g

15) Salted cod with mushrooms and mint

INGREDIENTS:

- ➤ 1/2 cup mushrooms (cleaned)
- ➤ 4 cherry tomatoes
- ➤ 7 ounces salted cod fillet (already soaked)
- ➤ Mint
- ➤ Oil
- ➤ Pine nuts
- ➤ Grated grana cheese

DIRECTIONS:

1. Sauté the mushrooms with the chopped cherry tomatoes and a little bit of water (season with salt, pepper and spices to taste).
2. Halfway through cooking, put the cod cut into bites to cook along with the mushrooms.
3. Add some chopped mint. In the meantime, blend in a mixer mint, pine nuts, oil, grana cheese (add salt to taste) until it reaches the consistency of a pesto.
4. Serve and enjoy by dipping the cod in the mint pesto.

NUTRITION:

Calories 168 Carbs 4g Fat 2g Protein 34g

16) Shrimp curry and dry Konjac rice

INGREDIENTS for 2 people:
- ➤ Red onion to taste
- ➤ ounces shrimps
- ➤ Extra virgin olive oil
- ➤ 1 cup thick coconut milk
- ➤ Curry to taste
- ➤ Konjac rice

DIRECTIONS:

1. In a nonstick pan, brown the onion with the oil.
2. Add the shrimps, stir and add the curry and coconut milk.
3. Let the sauce thicken over moderate heat.
4. Meanwhile, cook the Konjac rice for about 12 minutes.
5. Drain the rice and serve with the shrimps.

NUTRITION:

Calories 352 Carbs 17g Fat 20g Protein 26g

17) Shrimp risotto

INGREDIENTS:

- ➤ 1/2 cup low carb rice (such as Palmini)
- ➤ 1 tablespoon butter
- ➤ 1/4 cup cream cheese
- ➤ 1 dash cream (optional)
- ➤ Shrimps, already cooked

DIRECTIONS:

1. Melt the butter in a nonstick pan over medium heat.
2. Drain and rinse the rice with plenty of water. Add the rice to the melted butter and turn down to medium-low heat.
3. Add the cream cheese, dried chives, salt and pepper.
4. Stir until the cheese is melted (if you want to, add a dash of cream). Add shrimps at the last, mix and compose the dish.

NUTRITION:

Calories 359 Carbs 28g Fat 21g Protein 16g

18) Simmered sea bream

INGREDIENTS for 2 people:

- ➢ 2 sea breams
- ➢ Juice of half a lemon or a small lime (optional)
- ➢ Fresh or powdered ginger
- ➢ 1 garlic clove
- ➢ 2 onions
- ➢ 5 vine tomatoes
- ➢ 1 small green bell pepper (optional)
- ➢ 1 small yellow bell pepper (optional)
- ➢ Coriander to taste
- ➢ Oregano to taste
- ➢ Olive oil to taste
- ➢ Salt and pepper to taste

DIRECTIONS:

1. First of all, clean the fish and cut off the side fins (you can ask to do it at the fishmonger).
2. After that, season with salt, pepper and lemon, and let marinate. In the meantime, peel with a knife the tomatoes, clean and cut the onions and peppers into slices, cubes or as you want. Finely chop the ginger and garlic, heat a pan with oil and sauté the garlic for a minute.
3. Remove from the heat, add half of the ingredients all over the surface of the pan and lay the fish on top.
4. Cover the fish with the remaining ingredients, put the lid and let it cook for 20 minutes or until you see that the fish is cooked.
5. Uncover and add the finely chopped herbs. Let stand for a few minutes and you're done.
6. Tip: halfway through cooking, season with salt. If you see that the cooking lacks liquid, you can add water.
7. Remember that to make this recipe you can use any type of fish or the one you like best.

NUTRITION:

Calories 566 Carbs 58g Fat 14g Protein 53g

19) Spiced salmon en papillote

INGREDIENTS:

- ➢ ounces salmon fillet
- ➢ 1/2 chopped eggplant
- ➢ 1 zucchini
- ➢ 1 cherry tomato
- ➢ Chopped rosemary, sage, parsley and basil
- ➢ 2 green olives
- ➢ 1 tablespoon coconut oil

DIRECTIONS:

1. Place the salmon fillet in foil and add the other ingredients, all mixed with coconut oil.
2. Bake in the air fryer at 300° F (150° C) for 25 minutes.

NUTRITION:

Calories 251 Carbs 19g Fat 17g Protein 5g

20) Squid rings

INGREDIENTS:

- ➢ ounces squid rings
- ➢ 1 zucchini
- ➢ Extra virgin olive oil to taste
- ➢ Salt and pepper to taste
- ➢ Garlic powder to taste
- ➢ 1 Hass avocado

DIRECTIONS:

1. Cut the zucchini into rounds and brown them in a pan with plenty of extra virgin olive oil.
2. Add salt, pepper and garlic powder. After 5 minutes, add the squid rings and continue cooking over high heat for a few more minutes.
3. To make your meal even richer and tastier, serve with Haas avocado adding a drizzle of oil, salt and pepper to taste.

NUTRITION:

Calories 456 Carbs 10g Fat 32g Protein 32g

21) Squid soup

INGREDIENTS:

- 1 pound squid
- 3 celery sticks
- 1 red onion
- 1 garlic clove
- 1 pound fresh spinach
- Fresh chili pepper
- Tomato puree
- 1/2 glass white wine
- Extra virgin olive oil
- Salt

DIRECTIONS:

1. Cut the onion and celery into small cubes, and sauté them in a pan with the garlic clove and oil.
2. Now add the squid and sauté for 1 minute.
3. Over high heat, add the wine and salt to taste, put the lid on and cook for 15 minutes.
4. Add the tomato puree, chili pepper, spinach, put the lid on and cook for further 15 minutes.

NUTRITION:

Calories 530 Carbs 48g Fat 6g Protein 71g

22) Stuffed baked mussels

INGREDIENTS:

- 2 cups mussels (open)
- 1/2 cup almond flour
- 3/4 cup grated Parmesan cheese
- 1 egg
- Salt to taste
- Parsley to taste
- Spices to taste

DIRECTIONS:

1. Mix all the ingredients to create the filling and with the resulting mixture coat the mussels.
2. Arrange them in a baking sheet. Pour a drizzle of oil over the stuffed mussels and bake in the air fryer at 390° F (200° C) for 15 minutes.

NUTRITION:

Calories 665 Carbs 10g Fat 39g Protein 69g

23) Stuffed cuttlefishes

INGREDIENTS:

- 3 cuttlefishes
- 1/4 cup Parmesan cheese
- 1/2 cup almond flour
- 1 egg
- Parsley, pepper and garlic to taste
- Salt to taste
- Extra virgin olive oil to taste

DIRECTIONS:

1. Wash and clean the cuttlefishes. Cut the tentacles into small pieces and put them in a bowl with all the other ingredients, thus creating the filling.
2. Season with plenty of oil and cook in the air fryer at 355° F (180° C) for 10 minutes.

NUTRITION:

Calories 688 Carbs 7g Fat 23g Protein 114 g

14

VEGETABLES

1) Artichoke omelet with stretched-curd cheese

INGREDIENTS for 1 serving:

- ➢ 2 small eggs (3 ounces)
- ➢ 1/4 cup grated Parmesan cheese
- ➢ 1/4 cup stretched-curd cheese
- ➢ 1/2 cup frozen artichokes
- ➢ 1 tablespoon extra virgin olive oil
- ➢ 1 garlic clove
- ➢ Salt and pepper

DIRECTIONS:

1. Brown the artichokes with a little oil and garlic for about 10 minutes.
2. Chop them up and let them cool. In the meantime, combine all the other ingredients and finally add the artichokes.
3. Grease the baking sheet, sprinkle with Parmesan cheese and pour the mixture.
4. Bake in the oven at 355° F (180° C) for 20/25 minutes and enjoy.

NUTRITION:

Calories 509 Carbs 7g Fat 32g Protein 48g

2) Artichoke quiche

INGREDIENTS:

For the dough:

- ➢ 2 cups almond flour
- ➢ 1/2 cup sunflower seed flour
- ➢ 1/2 cup egg whites
- ➢ 1 tablespoon gomashio
- ➢ 1 1/2 tablespoons evo oil
- ➢ Thyme powder
- ➢ Rosemary powder

For the filling:

- ➢ 1/2 cup egg whites
- ➢ 3 tablespoons goat's milk ricotta
- ➢ 2 tablespoons Parmesan cheese
- ➢ Salt and pepper
- ➢ 4 artichokes

DIRECTIONS:

1. For the dough, mix all the ingredients until you get a compact mixture and let it stand for 5 minutes.
2. Roll out between 2 sheets of baking paper and line an 8-inch baking sheet with it.
3. Bake at 355° F (180° C) for 8 minutes.
4. For the filling, mix all the ingredients until you have a smooth mixture without lumps. Place it on the pre-cooked dough.
5. Cook the artichokes in wedges in the traditional way, that is with garlic, oil, parsley, salt and pepper.
6. You can also add a few hemp seeds. Add the artichokes to the quiche. Bake for another 25 minutes and then for 5 more in grill mode.

NUTRITION:

Calories 913 Carbs 22g Fat 65g Protein 60g

3) Asparagus omelet

INGREDIENTS:

- 2 cups asparagus
- 6 eggs
- 1/2 cup almond flour
- 3/4 cup grated Parmesan cheese
- 2 teaspoons salt
- Spices to taste

DIRECTIONS:

1. In a bowl, whisk together all the ingredients except the asparagus.
2. Pour the mixture into a greased baking sheet and arrange the asparagus on top of the mixture.
3. Bake at 390° F (200° C) for 15 minutes.

NUTRITION:

Calories 889 Carbs 17 Fat 59g Protein 73

4) Asparagus pinwheels

INGREDIENTS:

- 2 cups asparagus
- 6 eggs
- 3/4 cup grated Parmesan cheese
- 1 pinch baking soda
- 2 teaspoons salt
- Spices to taste
- Chopped mortadella to taste
- Chopped Gouda (or other cheese) to taste

DIRECTIONS:

1. In a bowl, whisk together all the ingredients except the asparagus, mortadella and Gouda.
2. Pour the mixture into a baking sheet lined with baking paper and place the asparagus, mortadella and Gouda on top of the mixture.
3. Bake at 390° F (200° C) for 15 minutes. Once the omelet has cooled down, roll it up with the help of the baking paper and cut it into many rounds.

NUTRITION:

Calories 824 Carbs 15g Fat 53g Protein 71g

5) Baked fennel

INGREDIENTS:

- 1 pound fennel
- 5 ounces turkey breast
- 1 cup mozzarella cheese
- Salt, olive oil and pepper to taste

DIRECTIONS:

4. Clean, wash and cut the fennel, then cook it in already salted boiling water for 15 minutes.
5. Drain and put it in a baking sheet lined with baking paper.
6. Make the first layer with the turkey breast and continue with the mozzarella cheese.
7. Drizzle with oil and bake in the preheated fan oven at 355° F (180° C) for 30 minutes or so (in grill mode during the last minutes).

NUTRITION:

Calories 643 Carbs 38g Fat 26g Protein 63g

6) Baked feta cheese with pumpkin, leek and pecans

INGREDIENTS:

- 1/2 pumpkin
- 2 leeks
- 1 garlic clove
- Feta cheese
- 1 cup pecans
- Oil, salt, pepper

DIRECTIONS:

1. Cut the pumpkin into cubes and the leek into slices. Include the green part of the leek which is delicious, but wash it well because there may be some soil.
2. Put the vegetables in a baking sheet, season with oil, salt and pepper and add a garlic clove for flavoring.
3. Bake at 390° F (200° C) for 15 minutes, then add 2/3 cup coarsely chopped pecans.
4. Stir the vegetables, create a hole in the middle for the feta and add the remaining whole pecans. Bake again for another 20 minutes.

NUTRITION:

Calories 941 Carbs 57g Fat 73g Protein 14g

7) Baked radicchio au gratin

INGREDIENTS for 2 people:

- ➤ 2/3 radicchio heads, depending on the size
- ➤ 2 packets Dièt Croc (snack made of spelt flour and linseeds)
- ➤ 1 garlic clove
- ➤ Plenty of fresh parsley
- ➤ Grated peel of 1 lemon
- ➤ Juice of 1/2 lemon
- ➤ 1 handful pine nuts or walnuts
- ➤ 2 tablespoons extra virgin olive oil
- ➤ 1 cup white vinegar
- ➤ Salt and pepper to taste

DIRECTIONS:

1. First, cut each head of radicchio into 4 parts and soak it in cold water with 1 cup of vinegar and 1 pinch of salt. Let stand for at least 1/2 hour.
2. In the meantime, prepare the lemon mixture by putting in the blender two packets of Dièt Croc, the grated peel of 1 lemon, plenty of parsley, 1 garlic clove (to taste) and the juice of 1/2 lemon.
3. Chop everything for a few moments. Then quickly dry the radicchio and place it on a baking sheet lined with baking paper, drizzle with 2 tablespoons of extra virgin olive oil and sprinkle with the lemon mixture.
4. Add the pine nuts or walnuts. Bake at 355° F (180° C) for 30 minutes or until desired browning and enjoy.

NUTRITION:

Calories 593 Carbs 11g Fat 52g Protein 21g

8) Baked stuffed peppers

INGREDIENTS:

- ➤ 6 fresh bell peppers
- ➤ 4 eggs
- ➤ 1/2 cup feta cheese
- ➤ Thyme and fresh oregano
- ➤ Salt and pepper
- ➤ Olives (optional)

DIRECTIONS:

1. First wash the peppers and cut off the top, remove the seeds, rinse and set aside.
2. In a bowl, break the eggs and season with salt, pepper, oregano and thyme.
3. Beat with a fork. Add the crumbled feta and, if necessary, the olives. Fill the peppers with the egg and feta mixture and cover each pepper with its own top.
4. Before baking, grease all the peppers with a little oil and salt and sprinkle some water over the baking sheet.
5. Bake at 355° F (180° C) for about 30 minutes. Check the cooking of both the eggs and the peppers.

NUTRITION:

Calories 652 Carbs 52g Fat 31g Protein 41g

9) Baked zucchini and egg "nests" with goat's milk cheese

INGREDIENTS:

- ➤ 2 large zucchinis
- ➤ 2 eggs
- ➤ 1/4 cup goat's milk cheese
- ➤ Extra virgin olive oil
- ➤ Salt and pepper to taste

DIRECTIONS:

1. Wash and dry the zucchinis. Using a spiral vegetable slicer, make zucchini noodles (zoodles).
2. Place them in a bowl and season with oil, salt and pepper.
3. Take a baking sheet covered with baking paper and arrange some "nests" with the zoodles, leaving space in the middle for the egg.
4. Crack the eggs and place them in the middle of each nest. Bake in preheated oven at 390° F (200° C) for about 20 minutes.
5. Remove from the oven, let cool slightly and add the goat's milk cheese in chunks. Season with salt and pepper.

NUTRITION:

Calories 444 Carbs 15g Fat 31g Protein 26g

10) Beet and chickpea hummus

INGREDIENTS:

- ➤ 1 1/2 cups cooked beet
- ➤ 1 cup cooked chickpeas
- ➤ 2 tablespoons extra virgin olive oil
- ➤ 1 tablespoon mustard
- ➤ 1/2 onion
- ➤ Juice of 1/2 lemon
- ➤ Sesame seeds to taste
- ➤ Pink salt to taste

DIRECTIONS:

1. Cook onion in boiling water until soft.

2. Put together all the ingredients and blend until you get a thick cream, garnish with sesame seeds and enjoy. You can also serve with a poached egg.

NUTRITION:

Calories 681 Carbs 78g Fat 33g Protein 20g

11) Broccoli and chlorophyll gnocchi

INGREDIENTS for 2 people:

- ➤ 2 1/2 cups blended cooked broccoli
- ➤ 3/4 cup grated Parmesan cheese (aged 30 months)
- ➤ 1 egg
- ➤ 1 scoop chlorophyll powder
- ➤ 1 tablespoon oat fiber
- ➤ 1 generous tablespoon psyllium
- ➤ Salt

DIRECTIONS:

1. Mix all ingredients together, shape small balls and create the classic
2. Italian gnocchi lines. Bake in a fan oven for 15 minutes at 320° F (160° C).
3. Cook in a pan with clarified butter and sage.

NUTRITION:

Calories 599 Carbs 38g Fat 30g Protein 43g

12) Broccoli and walnut velouté

INGREDIENTS:

- ➤ 1/2 sliced onion
- ➤ 1 garlic clove
- ➤ 6 cups broccoli
- ➤ 1/2 cup walnuts
- ➤ Extra virgin olive oil
- ➤ 3 tablespoons soy sauce
- ➤ Vegetable broth to taste

DIRECTIONS:

1. Sauté the onion and garlic in the oil. Add the broccoli, soy sauce and vegetable broth and bring to a boil.
2. When the broccoli is cooked, add the walnuts, salt to taste and blend.
3. Once plated, garnish with two walnuts and poppy seeds.

NUTRITION:

Calories 977 Carbs 74g Fat 58g Protein 41g

13) Broccoli cream with melted Asiago cheese and sausage chunks

INGREDIENTS for 1 serving:

- ➤ 3 cups broccoli
- ➤ 1 1/2 cups sugar-free almond milk
- ➤ 3 ounces chicken and turkey sausage
- ➤ 1 tablespoon extra virgin olive oil
- ➤ 1/4 cup PDO Asiago cheese
- ➤ 1/4 teaspoon xanthan gum
- ➤ Chopped parsley
- ➤ Chili pepper threads
- ➤ Salt and pepper to taste

DIRECTIONS:

1. Steam the broccoli florets or blanch them. In the meantime, brown the chopped sausage in a small pan.
2. Blend the broccoli with salt, pepper, milk and xanthan.
3. Boil for 5 minutes. Serve the obtained broccoli cream with sliced Asiago cheese, sausage chunks, parsley, and chili pepper threads.

NUTRITION:

Calories 465 Carbs 30g Fat 23g Protein 34g

14) Broccoli muffins

INGREDIENTS for 6 muffins:

- ➤ 2 eggs
- ➤ 1 cup egg whites
- ➤ Raw broccoli in pieces
- ➤ 1 tablespoon Parmesan cheese
- ➤ Salt and pepper to taste

DIRECTIONS:

1. Pour all the ingredients except broccoli into a bowl, mix with a fork and place in buttered molds.
2. Finally add the pieces of raw broccoli and bake at 355° F (180° C) for about 10 minutes.

NUTRITION:

Calories 314 Carbs 9g Fat 12g Protein 43g

15) Broccoli pie

INGREDIENTS:

- ➤ 3 eggs
- ➤ 2 tablespoons extra virgin olive oil
- ➤ 1/3 cup almond flour
- ➤ 2 cups broccoli
- ➤ Salt and garlic powder

DIRECTIONS:

1. First boil the broccoli and reduce it to a cream. Beat the egg whites until stiff.
2. Stir in the egg yolks, flour, salt and garlic powder. Finally add the broccoli cream.
3. Roll out the dough to obtain a thickness of about 1 inch.
4. Bake at 355° F (180° C) for 15/20 minutes. Once cooled, cut it into rectangles and stuff as you like, for example with ricotta and cherry tomatoes.

NUTRITION:

Calories 683 Carbs 19g Fat 54g Protein 30g

16) Broccoli soup with cheese

INGREDIENTS:

- ➤ 2 cups broccoli, cut into florets
- ➤ 1 cup Swiss cheese flakes (such as Edam)
- ➤ 1/2 cup cream
- ➤ 2 cups vegetable broth
- ➤ 1 garlic clove, minced
- ➤ 1 tablespoon olive oil

DIRECTIONS:

1. Heat the oil in a deep pan and sauté the garlic for one minute.
2. Add the broth, broccoli and cream and let cook slowly for 15 minutes.
3. Finally, add the cheese flakes and let melt while stirring continuously.

NUTRITION:

Calories 972 Carbs 36g Fat 70g Protein 50g

17) Brussels sprout clafoutis

INGREDIENTS:

- ➤ 1 1/2 pounds Brussels sprout
- ➤ 4 eggs
- ➤ 3/4 cup fresh cream
- ➤ 2/3 cup Emmental cheese, julienned
- ➤ Salt and pepper

DIRECTIONS:

1. Steam the sprouts, keeping them al dente. Put them in a baking sheet and add the eggs mixed with all the other ingredients.
2. Bake in the fan oven at 390° F (200° C) for 20 minutes until golden brown.

NUTRITION:

Calories 1218 Carbs 23g Fat 98g Protein 61g

18) Cabbage and tuna salad

INGREDIENTS:

- ➤ 1/4 cabbage
- ➤ 5 ounces tuna
- ➤ 1/2 avocado
- ➤ Juice of 1/2 lemon
- ➤ 1 teaspoon mustard
- ➤ 1 teaspoon mayonnaise
- ➤ Salt and pepper to taste

DIRECTIONS:

1. Thinly slice the cabbage. Chop the avocado into small pieces.
2. In a small bowl, mix the mustard, mayonnaise, lemon juice, salt and pepper.
3. In a bowl, put the cabbage, avocado and tuna, pour the previous mixture and stir. Serve and enjoy.

NUTRITION:

Calories 383 Carbs 8g Fat 26g Protein 30g

19) Carrot rolls

INGREDIENTS:

For the base:

- ➢ 4 eggs
- ➢ 2 tablespoons Parmesan cheese
- ➢ 1 cup grated carrot (1 medium-sized carrot)
- ➢ Salt and pepper
- ➢ 1 tablespoon turmeric

For the filling:

- ➢ 2/3 cup fresh cream cheese
- ➢ Bresaola or ham
- ➢ Grana cheese
- ➢ Arugula or spinach

DIRECTIONS:

1. In a bowl, break the eggs and beat them with the Parmesan cheese, salt, grated carrot and turmeric.
2. Bake in the static oven at 355° F (180° C) for 10/15 minutes in a rectangular baking sheet.
3. Once the base is cooked, top it with cheese, ham or bresaola and spinach or arugula, depending on your taste.
4. Roll it up. Let stand the roll in the fridge for at least 1 hour.

NUTRITION:

Calories 904 Carbs 29g Fat 54g Protein 75g

20) Cauliflower bites

INGREDIENTS:

- ➢ 1 medium-sized cauliflower
- ➢ Grated ginger to taste
- ➢ Parsley to taste
- ➢ Salt
- ➢ Pepper
- ➢ 1 tablespoon clarified butter or coconut oil

DIRECTIONS:

1. Clean the cauliflower, wash and dry it. Break it up to create bite-sized pieces.
2. Place them in a bowl with coconut oil or clarified butter, salt, pepper, grated ginger and parsley.
3. Mix and place on a baking sheet lined with baking paper.

4. Bake in the hot fan oven at 355° F (180° C) for about 30 minutes. Finish cooking in grill mode for another 15 minutes. Serve and enjoy.

NUTRITION:

Calories 162 Carbs 7g Fat 14g Protein 2g

21) Cauliflower couscous

INGREDIENTS:

- ➢ 1 1/3 pounds cauliflower
- ➢ Brussels sprouts
- ➢ Leek
- ➢ 1 garlic clove
- ➢ 2 tablespoons pitted olives
- ➢ Fresh cherry tomatoes
- ➢ 1 pomegranate
- ➢ Fresh parsley
- ➢ Extra virgin olive oil
- ➢ Salt
- ➢ Chili pepper
- ➢ Lemon juice

DIRECTIONS:

1. Remove the leaves and detach the florets from the cauliflower.
2. Rinse them under fresh running water, dry them with kitchen paper and blend them, a few at a time, in a food processor.
3. Then transfer the obtained cauliflower grains in a bowl.
4. Fry the garlic and leek together with the chopped olives.
5. Add the halved cherry tomatoes and Brussels sprouts previously blanched over high heat.
6. Pour in the cauliflower grains and stir, season with salt and add chili pepper and chopped parsley. Finally turn off the heat and add a little lemon juice, a drizzle of olive oil and the pomegranate grains.

NUTRITION:

Calories 531 Carbs 70g Fat 22g Protein 13g

22) Cauliflower cutlet

INGREDIENTS:

- ➤ 1 cauliflower
- ➤ 2 eggs
- ➤ Hazelnut flour to taste for breading

DIRECTIONS:

1. Wash, clean and dry the cauliflower, and cut it into not too thin slices.
2. Beat the eggs with salt and pepper. As with traditional cutlets, dip the cauliflower slices into the egg and then into the flour, pressing well on all sides. Bake in the air fryer at 390° F (200° C) for 20 minutes.

NUTRITION:

Calories 170 Carbs 6g Fat 10g Protein 15g

23) Cauliflower gateau

INGREDIENTS:

For the base:

- ➤ 2 pounds steamed cauliflower
- ➤ 1/3 cup butter
- ➤ 1/2 cup fresh cream
- ➤ 4 large eggs
- ➤ Parmesan cheese
- ➤ Parsley
- ➤ Salt, pepper

For the filling:

- ➤ Mozzarella cheese
- ➤ Cooked ham

DIRECTIONS:

1. First, mash the steamed cauliflower with a potato masher.
2. Add the remaining ingredients and mix. Roll out in a buttered baking sheet and sprinkle with keto breadcrumbs.
3. Add the mozzarella cheese and cooked ham and cover with the remaining dough. Sprinkle with some breadcrumbs mixed with Parmesan cheese. Baked in the hot oven at 355° F (180° C) for about 40 minutes.

NUTRITION:

Calories 1343 Carbs 27g Fat 112g Protein 58g

24) Cauliflower hummus

INGREDIENTS:

- ➤ 1/2 cauliflower
- ➤ 1 garlic clove
- ➤ 1 teaspoon salt
- ➤ 2 tablespoons extra virgin olive oil
- ➤ Paprika
- ➤ Chives

DIRECTIONS:

1. First boil the cauliflower and put it in the blender (you can also use the hand blender).
2. Season with salt, oil and garlic, and blend until you get a cream.
3. Put it in a container and finish with more oil, chives and paprika.

NUTRITION:

Calories 272 Carbs 4g Fat 28g Protein 1g

25) Cauliflower pizza

INGREDIENTS for 1 person:

For the base:

- ➤ 1/2 cup cauliflower
- ➤ 1/2 cup grated Parmesan cheese
- ➤ 2 tablespoons grated Gouda cheese
- ➤ 1 egg
- ➤ 1 pinch salt
- ➤ 1/2 teaspoon oregano

For the filling:

- ➤ 1/4 cup tomato puree
- ➤ 1 ounce raw ham
- ➤ 1/4 cup grated mozzarella cheese

DIRECTIONS:

1. For the base, finely chop the cauliflower and mix with the Parmesan cheese, Gouda, egg, salt and oregano.
2. Spread on a baking sheet lined with baking paper and bake at 390° F (200° C) for 10 minutes.
3. Pour the tomato puree, top with raw ham and mozzarella and bake for another 10 minutes at 390° F (200° C).

NUTRITION:

Calories 518 Carbs 12g Fat 35g Protein 40g

26) Cauliflower puree with salmon

INGREDIENTS:

- 1 small cauliflower
- 2 tablespoons cream
- 2 tablespoons grated Parmesan cheese
- Nutmeg
- Salt and pepper
- Salmon
- Sesame seeds

DIRECTIONS:

1. Boil the cauliflower and blend it with all the other ingredients.
2. Garnish the puree with some salmon and sesame seeds.

NUTRITION:

Calories 320 Carbs 7g Fat 18g Protein 34g

27) Cauliflower rice

INGREDIENTS for 2 people:

- 1 pound cauliflower (frozen)
- 3 ounces bacon, diced
- Olive oil
- Spices to taste

DIRECTIONS:

1. Blend the ingredients in the mixer for a few seconds.
2. Cook the mixture in a pan with extra virgin olive oil over very high heat for about 6 minutes.
3. Meanwhile, sauté the bacon cubes. Add salt and spices to taste.
4. Cook for about 6 more minutes, add the bacon and enjoy.

NUTRITION:

Calories 276 Carbs 8g Fat 20g Protein 16g

28) Cauliflower risotto with crispy Jerusalem artichoke

INGREDIENTS for 3 people:

- 5 cups cauliflower
- 1/4 cup Jerusalem artichoke
- 1/4 red onion
- 1/4 cup white wine
- 1 1/2 tablespoons butter
- 2 tablespoons Parmesan cheese
- Parsley
- Extra virgin olive oil
- Salt and pepper

DIRECTIONS:

1. After washing and slicing the Jerusalem artichoke, fry it in oil over very low heat (when it is almost cooked, slightly turn up the heat).
2. Then finely chop the onion and a small piece of Jerusalem artichoke and sauté in the same pan, with the same oil.
3. Wash, dry and blend the cauliflower and add to the sauteed mixture. Let cook a little, then pour in some wine and cook with the lid on for about 12/15 minutes.
4. Add the butter, turn off the heat and cover again.
5. Add the Parmesan cheese and parsley, mix, drizzle with oil, serve and lay the crispy Jerusalem artichoke on top.

NUTRITION:

Calories 450 Carbs 39g Fat 26g Protein 15g

29) Cauliflower "volcano"

INGREDIENTS:

- One medium-sized cauliflower
- 2 tablespoons butter
- 1 teaspoon minced garlic
- 1/2 cup grated Parmesan cheese
- 2 1/2 ounces bacon
- Salt, pepper and olive oil for seasoning
- Arugula

DIRECTIONS:

1. Wash the cauliflower, cut it into florets or simply into pieces. Boil in a pot with salted water for about 10 minutes (until very tender).
2. Meanwhile, sauté the bacon. When the cauliflower is cooked, transfer it into the food processor, add the butter, garlic, Parmesan cheese, salt and pepper. Blend until smooth (1-2 minutes).
3. Add the bacon and arugula as a side dish. Serve immediately.

NUTRITION:

Calories 440 Carbs 11g Fat 30g Protein 32g

30) Chard and broccoli savory pie

INGREDIENTS:

- Chard and broccoli
- 1/2 cup grated Asiago cheese
- 1/4 cup butter
- 1 cup shredded coconut
- 2/3 cup seed flour
- 1 egg
- Salt to taste

DIRECTIONS:

1. Prepare the dough with all the ingredients at room temperature, then let stand for 20/30 minutes in the fridge.
2. Roll out in an 8 inch cake pan lined with baking paper and bake in the oven at 355° F (180° C) for 15 minutes.
3. In the meantime, prepare the filling with the vegetables you prefer, blanched in water (as with chard and broccoli) or stir-fried (in the case of mushrooms and zucchini) depending on your taste.
4. Mix with an egg, cheese to taste (in this case ricotta) and spices such as nutmeg or herbs.
5. Put back in the oven and bake until the filling is firm. You can also top with a bit of mozzarella or other stretched-curd cheese to make a crispy crust.

NUTRITION:

Calories 787 Carbs 14g Fat 72g Protein 20g

31) Creamy broccoli with coconut and curry

INGREDIENTS:

- 5 cups broccoli
- 1/2 onion
- 1 cup coconut cream
- Salt and pepper to taste
- 1 teaspoon curry powder

DIRECTIONS:

1. Place the broccoli and sliced onion in the slow cooker, mix the coconut cream with the salt, pepper and curry powder, then pour the mixture over the broccoli.
2. Cook on high mode for 2 1/2 hours.

NUTRITION:

Calories 644 Carbs 47g Fat 43g Protein 19g

32) Fennel and leek velouté

INGREDIENTS:

- 7 ounces fennel
- 2 ounces leeks
- Bone broth for cooking
- Salt and pepper
- 1/4 cup coconut cream for blending
- Spices (curry, garlic sauce, parsley)
- 1 tablespoon of apple cider vinegar (optional)

DIRECTIONS:

1. Cook the vegetables in the broth over low heat until soft.
2. Once cooked, if there is too much broth, you can remove some.
3. Add the coconut cream and spices. Blend everything together, serve and add mixed seeds to taste (pumpkin, sunflower, sesame, poppy).

NUTRITION:

Calories 403 Carbs 55g Fat 16g Protein 10g

33) Gluten-free carrot plum cake

INGREDIENTS:

- 1 cup rice flour
- 1 sachet organic yeast
- 2 eggs
- 1/4 cup egg whites
- 1/2 cup erythritol (or coconut/cane sugar)
- 2 1/3 cups grated carrots
- 1/2 cup olive oil

DIRECTIONS:

1. In blender put the carrots, erythritol, eggs, egg whites and oil, and mix. Sift the flour and baking powder, add in the blender and blend again.
2. Pour the mixture into a plum cake mold and bake in the static oven at 355° F (180° C) for 40 minutes.
3. You can top with low carb almond cream with no added sugar by Revolution03.

NUTRITION:

Calories 1028 Carbs 159g Fat 27g Protein 38g

34) Gnudi (Tuscan spinach and ricotta dumplings)

INGREDIENTS:

- 6 cups spinach (fresh or frozen)
- 1 cup Parmesan cheese
- 2 cups robiola cheese
- 2 eggs
- 2 tablespoon bamboo fiber
- 1 tablespoon xanthan
- Sage
- Nutmeg
- Salt and pepper

DIRECTIONS:

1. Cook the spinach in a pan with a drizzle of oil for about 10 minutes. Once cooled, squeeze very well.
2. Add the eggs, cheese, chopped sage, salt and pepper, Parmesan cheese and fibers (xanthan and bamboo).
3. Mix with the help of a blender. Shape small balls and crush them between your hands.
4. Bake in the static oven at 355° F (180° C) for 10 minutes. Serve hot and topped with butter, sage and Parmesan cheese.
5.

NUTRITION:

Calories 1292 Carbs 66g Fat 74g Protein 91g

35) Green beans with almonds

INGREDIENTS:

- ➤ 2 cups green beans
- ➤ 1/2 cup almond milk
- ➤ Salt and garlic powder to taste
- ➤ 1/2 tablespoon olive oil

DIRECTIONS:

1. Grease the slow cooker with oil and put all the ingredients in it.
2. Cook over high heat for 2 hours.
3. Before serving, garnish with almond slivers.

NUTRITION:

Calories 212 Carbs 16g Fat 15g Protein 4g

36) Half-moon stuffed with broccoli rabe

INGREDIENTS:

For the dough:

- ➤ 1/3 cup grated mozzarella cheese for pizza
- ➤ 1/3 cup almond flour
- ➤ 1/4 cup cream cheese
- ➤ 1 egg

For the filling:

- ➤ 3 cups frozen broccoli rabe
- ➤ Extra virgin olive oil
- ➤ Garlic
- ➤ 4 anchovies
- ➤ Pitted black olives
- ➤ Capers

DIRECTIONS:

1. Melt the cheeses in a bain-marie or in the microwave, then add the almond flour and egg.
2. Make a homogeneous dough with your hands. Spread it on a baking sheet covered with baking paper and bake for about 8 minutes at 390° F (200 ° C).
3. In the meantime, fry the garlic in the extra virgin olive oil and add the broccoli rabe.
4. Let it cook for at least 5 minutes and add the remaining ingredients.
5. Do not add salt, the ingredients are already quite salty.
6. Take the dough out of the oven and pour the filling over one half, folding the other half to form a half-moon. Bake for another 12 minutes or so.

NUTRITION:

Calories 584 Carbs 17g Fat 46g Protein 27g

37) Keto baked omelet with vegetables

INGREDIENTS:

- ➤ 4 eggs
- ➤ 2 tablespoons bamboo flour
- ➤ 1/4 cup speck cubes
- ➤ 1/2 cup milk (almond, coconut or cow)
- ➤ 1/4 onion
- ➤ 1/4 cup grana cheese
- ➤ Salt and pepper
- ➤ Spinach
- ➤ Zucchini
- ➤ Broccoli

DIRECTIONS:

1. Blanch all the vegetables individually and cut them into small pieces (no need to cook them too much). In a bowl beat the eggs, salt, pepper and the bamboo flour that will make the omelet soft.
2. Add the finely chopped bacon and onion, Parmesan cheese and milk.
3. In a plum cake mold lined with baking paper, place the vegetables in layers and pour the egg mixture over them.
4. Bake at 355° F (180° C) for about 20/25 minutes.

NUTRITION:

Calories 688 Carbs 7g Fat 44g Protein 66g

38) Keto Brussels sprouts, eggs and Parmesan cheese

INGREDIENTS for 2 servings:

- ➤ For the base:
- ➤ 1 1/2 cups brussels sprouts
- ➤ 4 eggs
- ➤ For the fondue:
- ➤ 2 tablespoons clarified butter
- ➤ 1 tablespoon mascarpone cheese
- ➤ 1 tablespoon coconut flour
- ➤ 1/2 cup Parmesan cheese
- ➤ 1/2 cup plant milk

DIRECTIONS:

1. Wash the brussels sprouts and cut them in half, place them in a baking sheet and season with oil and salt.
2. Add a little water. Bake at 355° F (180° C) for 20 minutes.
3. Meanwhile, prepare the fondue. In a small pan, melt the butter and mascarpone cheese, add flour, Parmesan cheese and milk, mix until creamy, add salt and pepper to taste.
4. Arrange the fondue on the bottom of a baking sheet and the sprouts on top leaving some holes to break the eggs in. Bake for 10 minutes at 375° F (190° C).

NUTRITION:

Calories 959 Carbs 26g Fat 70g Protein 56g

39) Keto fennel au gratin

INGREDIENTS:

- ➢ 2 fennels
- ➢ 1 cup mascarpone cheese
- ➢ Parmesan cheese

DIRECTIONS:

1. Clean and cut the fennel into thin slices. Steam and add salt to taste.
2. Once cooked, melt the mascarpone cheese in a small pan and pour it over the fennel.
3. Add Parmesan cheese and plenty of chopped fresh sage. Bake in the hot oven at 390° F (200° C) until golden brown.

NUTRITION:

Calories 739 Carbs 14g Fat 71g Protein 11g

40) Keto gazpacho (Spanish soup of raw, blended vegetables)

INGREDIENTS:

- ➢ 5 fairly ripe cherry tomatoes
- ➢ 1/4 cup bell pepper
- ➢ 1/2 avocado
- ➢ Juice of 1/2 lime + 1 slice for garnish
- ➢ 1 cucumber
- ➢ 4 tablespoons extra virgin olive oil
- ➢ 1 tablespoon MCT oil
- ➢ Salt and white pepper
- ➢ Garlic powder

DIRECTIONS:

1. Blend everything together, garnish with a slice of lime and your favorite herbs, and finally drizzle with oil.

NUTRITION:

Calories 679 Carbs 7g Fat 71g Protein 4g

41) Keto poke bowl with tofu

INGREDIENTS:

For the base:

- ➢ 2 cups spinach
- ➢ 1 tablespoon chili peppers stuffed with tuna
- ➢ 1/2 cup soybean sprouts
- ➢ 1/4 cup common mushrooms
- ➢ 1/4 cup bell peppers
- ➢ 1/4 cup organic tofu
- ➢ 2 tablespoons soy sauce

For the sauce:

- ➢ 2 tablespoons mayonnaise
- ➢ 1 1/2 tablespoons Greek yogurt 5%
- ➢ Plant milk to taste

DIRECTIONS:

1. For the base, slice the mushrooms and cook them in a pan with extra virgin olive oil and garlic.
2. Slice the tofu and cook with a little soy sauce. Let it toast on both sides.
3. Clean and cut the peppers, cook them in a pan or in the air fryer. Put everything together in the dish.
4. For the sauce, mix the mayonnaise and Greek yogurt. To make it more fluid, add a little bit of plant milk.

NUTRITION:

Calories 566 Carbs 44g Fat 28g Protein 35g

42) Leeks au gratin

INGREDIENTS:

- 6 leeks
- 1/2 cup cooked ham
- Cooking cream
- Grana cheese

DIRECTIONS:

1. Boil the leeks in large chunks for about 10 minutes, then cut them in half lengthwise.
2. In a baking sheet, put a thin layer of cream and arrange half of the leeks with salt and pepper, then add the chopped ham, a little cream and some grated Grana cheese.
3. Make a second layer in the same way and bake at 355° F (180° C) for about 20 minutes.

NUTRITION:

Calories 560 Carbs 78g Fat 15g Protein 28g

43) Low-carb zucchini fettuccine pasta with feta cheese and zucchini pesto, fresh basil, walnuts and sunflower seeds

INGREDIENTS for 2 people:

- 1/2 clove garlic
- 1 tuft basil (approx. 1 cup)
- 3/4 tablespoon walnuts
- 1 tablespoon sunflower seeds
- 3 light green zucchinis (about 2 cups) (do not use those zucchinis with dark green watery peels, they ruin the dish!)
- 3 tablespoons extra virgin olive oil
- 1/2 cup feta or light feta cheese
- 1 generous tablespoon grated Parmesan cheese (or brewer's yeast flakes for a vegan version)
- Salt and pepper to taste

DIRECTIONS:

1. Peel the garlic and pull off the basil leaves.

Cut lengthwise 2 and a half zucchinis into very thin slices with a peeler or mandoline.

2. Brown the sunflower seeds and walnuts in a nonstick pan for a few seconds without burning until they release a toasted aroma.
3. Blend the toasted nuts and seeds together with the garlic, basil, the remaining half of the zucchini cut into pieces, a pinch of salt,
4. Parmesan cheese (or yeast) and drizzled oil. Operate the blender intermittently until you get a homogenous but somewhat coarse pesto.
5. Place the zucchini fettuccine on plates. Sprinkle with a little lemon juice, pepper and salt. Break the feta cheese with your hands and distribute it on the zucchini. Dress with the pesto.

NUTRITION:

Calories 848 Carbs 24g Fat 70g Protein 30g

44) Onion, zucchini and smoked scamorza omelet

INGREDIENTS:

- Tropea onions
- 1 zucchini
- 1 slice smoked scamorza cheese
- 4 eggs
- Parsley
- Salt and pepper to taste
- 2 tablespoons ghee (clarified butter) or extra virgin olive oil

DIRECTIONS:

1. Slice the Tropea onions and sauté them in a pan with hot oil.
2. Check them often so they don't burn. In the meantime, cut the zucchini into rounds and add them to the onions.
3. Cook for a few minutes over medium-high heat.
4. Cut the smoked scamorza into thin slices. Beat the eggs with salt, pepper and parsley.
5. At this point, turn up the heat and add the beaten eggs to the cooking vegetables.

NUTRITION:

Calories 767 Carbs 15g Fat 55g Protein 54g

45) Pumpkin focaccia bread

INGREDIENTS:

- ➤ 1 cup cooked and blended pumpkin pulp
- ➤ 2 cups RevoMix Pizza flour by Revolution03
- ➤ 2/3 cup cold water
- ➤ 2 tablespoons seed oil
- ➤ 1/2 teaspoon salt
- ➤ Rosemary

DIRECTIONS:

1. In a bowl, pour the RevoMix flour with the salt and add the cold water in the middle, beginning to mix with a fork.
2. At this point, add the pumpkin and little by little also the seed oil, starting to knead with your hands.
3. Let the dough stand, covered with plastic wrap, for 45 minutes.
4. After that, roll out the dough in a baking sheet and let it rise, covered, for about 1 hour. Brush the surface with olive oil and press with your fingers to form the characteristic focaccia holes.
5. Season with rosemary and coarse salt. Bake in the static preheated oven at 355° F (180° C) for 25 minutes.

NUTRITION:

Calories 453 Carbs 14g Fat 18g Protein 59g

46) Pumpkin tart

INGREDIENTS:

For the dough:
- ➤ 3/4 cup hazelnut flour
- ➤ 1/3 cup chufa flour
- ➤ 1/3 cup coconut flour
- ➤ 2 egg whites
- ➤ 2 tablespoons extra virgin olive oil
- ➤ Salt

For the filling:
- ➤ 4 cups pumpkin, cut into very small cubes
- ➤ Oregano
- ➤ Thyme
- ➤ Rosemary
- ➤ Chives
- ➤ Olive oil
- ➤ Strips of smoked bacon
- ➤ 2 tablespoons almond milk
- ➤ Parmesan cheese
- ➤ Salt

DIRECTIONS:

1. For the dough, mix all the flours with salt, add the egg whites, oil and knead until you get a compact dough.
2. Let it stand in the fridge for 30 minutes.
3. For the filling, season in a bowl the pumpkin cubes with all the flavorings, oil and salt.
4. Place in a baking sheet lined with baking paper and bake at 390° F (200° C) until golden brown.
5. Brown the bacon and add it to the pumpkin. Lay the dough on a 10-inch baking sheet in the shape of a tart, place the pumpkin on top along with the egg whites mixed with 1 tablespoon of almond milk and 3 tablespoons of Parmesan cheese.
6. Bake at 430° F (220° C) for 20 minutes.

NUTRITION:

Calories 1343 Carbs 67g Fat 99g Protein 45g

47) Radicchio, gorgonzola cheese and walnuts

INGREDIENTS for 2 people:

- ➢ 2 plants of long red radicchio
- ➢ 3/4 cup gorgonzola cheese (sweet or spicy)
- ➢ 6 walnuts
- ➢ 4 tablespoons extra virgin olive oil
- ➢ Black pepper to taste
- ➢ Salt to taste

DIRECTIONS:

1. Remove the outer leaves of the radicchio, rinse it and divide it into 4 slices (cutting lengthwise).
2. Line a baking sheet with baking paper and place the radicchio slices slightly spaced. Add a drizzle of oil, salt and pepper to taste.
3. Bake for 20 minutes in a fan oven with grill at 390° F (200° C).
4. While waiting, shell the walnuts and chop them coarsely (even with the help of a blender).
5. Once baked in the oven, place the gorgonzola cheese on each radicchio slice while it is still hot (to melt it and create a sort of icing).
6. To complete the recipe, add the chopped walnuts and serve.

NUTRITION:

Calories 1009 Carbs 13g Fat 95g Protein 26g

48) Red cabbage burger

INGREDIENTS:

- ➢ 2 cups red cabbage
- ➢ 2 eggs
- ➢ Salt
- ➢ Pepper
- ➢ 1 generous tablespoon psyllium

DIRECTIONS:

1. Blend everything together and with the help of a spoon place the mixture in a hot nonstick pan.
2. Gently turn between cooking one side and the other.

NUTRITION:

Calories 234 Carbs 21g Fat 10g Protein 15g

49) Red pumpkin parmigiana

INGREDIENTS:

- ➢ 2 pounds pumpkin (weight with skin)
- ➢ 2 cups mozzarella or provola cheese
- ➢ 5 ounces cooked ham
- ➢ Extra virgin olive oil
- ➢ Parmesan cheese to taste
- ➢ Almond flour to taste
- ➢ Salt

DIRECTIONS:

1. Remove the seeds and the skin from the pumpkin and cut it with a knife into thin slices (maximum 5 mm). Cover them with almond flour.
2. Brush a baking sheet with a little oil. Make a layer of pumpkin, sprinkle with Parmesan cheese, cooked ham, sliced mozzarella, a little oil and a pinch of salt.
3. Continue like this until all ingredients are well combined.
4. Finish with pumpkin slices, Parmesan cheese, a sprinkle of almond flour, oil, salt and a pinch of pepper. Bake in the preheated oven at 390° F (200° C) for 20 minutes.
5. Continue cooking until a crust forms. Let cool and serve. It is delicious both hot and at room temperature.

NUTRITION:

Calories 1127 Carbs 75g Fat 54g Protein 86g

50) Ricotta cheese medallions with crispy spinach and cream of gorgonzola and walnuts

INGREDIENTS for 2 people:

- 14 ounces spinach
- Butter
- For the medallions:
- 2/3 cup ricotta cheese
- 1 egg
- 1 tablespoon Parmesan cheese
- Salt
- For the gorgonzola cream:
- 1/3 cup cream
- 1/3 cup gorgonzola cheese
- 1/4 cup walnuts

DIRECTIONS:

1. First prepare the gorgonzola cream by heating the cream in a pan until it comes to a boil, then add the gorgonzola and walnuts.
2. Let everything mix together, blend and set aside.
3. Prepare the spinach (fresh or frozen) by drying it in a pan with some salt.
4. At the end of the cooking, add some butter and set aside.
5. Make the medallions by putting together all the listed ingredients and with the help of a ring mold give the proper shape.
6. Cook in a pan with a little oil, garlic and mint. Let cook on both sides until it forms a light crust.
7. Put everything in the plate: spinach, medallion, cream and some chopped walnuts. Enjoy hot.

NUTRITION:

Calories 745 Carbs 26g Fat 53g Protein 43g

51) Roasted asparagus with almonds

INGREDIENTS:

- 1 bunch large/medium-sized asparagus
- Olive oil to taste
- Salt and pepper to taste
- 1 tablespoon flaked almonds
- A few leaves arugula

DIRECTIONS:

1. Clean the asparagus. Season with oil and herbs.
2. You can cook it in the oven at 355° F (180° C) for 20/25 minutes, in the air fryer at the same temperature for 10 minutes or in a greased and preheated steak pan for 15 minutes.
3. Turn halfway through cooking and season with almonds and arugula.

NUTRITION:

Calories 603 Carbs 6g Fat 62g Protein 5g

52) Sauerkraut, radish and chicken soup with sour cream

INGREDIENTS for 2 people:

- 1/2 onion
- 1 garlic clove
- 1/2 celery stick
- 5 or 6 radishes
- ounces chicken breast fillets cut into small cubes
- 1 pinch ground cumin or cumin seeds
- 2 cups hot vegetable broth
- 1 cup ready-made sauerkrauts
- 1 tablespoon olive oil
- 1 sprig parsley
- 2 tablespoons sour cream or whole Greek yoghurt
- Salt and pepper

DIRECTIONS:

1. Peel the onion and garlic and chop them into small pieces.
2. Slice the celery and radishes. In a pan, place the oil, chicken cut in very small pieces, onion and garlic, celery, radishes and cumin.
3. Sauté over medium heat for about 10 minutes.
4. Add the hot vegetable broth, sauerkrauts, a pinch of salt and pepper and stir.
5. Let come to a boil and simmer for about 10 minutes. In the meantime, chop the parsley. Serve the soup and garnish with parsley and a spoonful of sour cream.

NUTRITION:

Calories 534 Carbs 9g Fat 29g Protein 60g

53) Spelt couscous with turmeric, peas, carrots and zucchini

INGREDIENTS for 1 person:

- 1/2 cup whole spelt couscous
- 1/2 cup water
- Turmeric and salt to taste
- 1/2 cup frozen peas
- 1 carrot
- 1 zucchini
- 1 tablespoon olive oil

DIRECTIONS:

1. Bring the water to a boil, turn off the heat and add the turmeric and 1 pinch of salt. Pour in the couscous and let stand for 5-7 minutes with the lid on.
2. Add 1 tablespoon of oil and shake with a fork. Sauté the diced vegetables with the peas.
3. Serve the couscous with the sautéed vegetables.

NUTRITION:

Calories 385 Carbs 49g Fat 15g Protein 13g

54) Spinach and ricotta pinwheels

INGREDIENTS:

For the base:

- ➤ 1 cup almond flour
- ➤ 1/4 cup Parmesan cheese
- ➤ 1/4 cup extra virgin olive oil
- ➤ 1 tablespoon instant yeast
- ➤ 1 egg
- ➤ 1 teaspoon xanthan gum
- ➤ 1 teaspoon salt
- ➤ Spices to taste
- ➤ For the filling:
- ➤ cups spinach
- ➤ 1/2 cup ricotta cheese
- ➤ Salt to taste
- ➤ Garlic powder to taste
- ➤ Extra virgin olive oil to taste

DIRECTIONS:

1. For the filling, sauté the spinach with oil, salt and garlic powder over medium heat.
2. Once cooked, turn off the heat, gently add the ricotta cheese and let cool.
3. For the base, mix all the ingredients and pour the mixture between two sheets of baking paper giving it a rectangular shape.
4. Stuff with the filling and roll up with the help of the baking paper.
5. Bake the whole roll covered with baking paper in the preheated oven at 390° F (200° C) for 15 minutes. Once cooked, let cool and cut out the pinwheels.

NUTRITION:

Calories 704 Carbs 25g Fat 48g Protein 44g

55) Spinach gnocchi

INGREDIENTS:

- ➤ 14 ounces frozen spinach
- ➤ 2 tablespoons lupin flour
- ➤ 2 tablespoons coconut flour
- ➤ Salt and pepper
- ➤ 2 tablespoons butter
- ➤ Garlic
- ➤ Parmesan cheese

DIRECTIONS:

1. Dry the spinach in a pan (you can use fresh spinach too). You will need to get rid of ALL the water (salt can help).
2. Let cool in a bowl and then add the flours. Mix first with a fork and then with your hands until you get a smooth and homogeneous dough.
3. Shape small balls and press them slightly with a fork to give the classic gnocchi shape.
4. Lightly toast some garlic with butter in a pan, pour in the gnocchi and a little pepper.
5. Wait just enough time, so that the liquid is absorbed and a light crust forms.
6. Serve, drizzle with oil and sprinkle with plenty of Parmesan cheese.

NUTRITION:

Calories 389 Carbs 28g Fat 22g Protein 19g

56) Spinach muffins

INGREDIENTS for 5 muffins:

- ➢ 5 cups (1 pound bag) fresh spinach
- ➢ 3 tablespoons grated Parmesan cheese
- ➢ 1/3 cup cream cheese
- ➢ 1 1/2 ounces cooked ham
- ➢ 1/2 cup egg whites
- ➢ 2 basil leaves, chopped
- ➢ 5 walnuts
- ➢ Salt, pepper, nutmeg to taste

DIRECTIONS:

1. Boil the spinach, let cool and squeeze to remove as much liquid as possible.
2. Then put it into a bowl along with the Parmesan and cream cheese and begin to mix.
3. Add half of the coarsely chopped walnuts, the basil and the ham cut into strips and continue to knead.
4. Finally, add the egg whites, salt and seasoning. Pour the mixture into the muffin mold and cook in the microwave at 450 W for 7 minutes.
5. Take the muffins out of the mold by turning them upside down and sprinkle with Parmesan cheese. Enjoy cold.

NUTRITION:

Calories 688 Carbs 55g Fat 24g Protein 62g

57) Spinach pie

INGREDIENTS:

- ➢ 1 cup almond flour
- ➢ 1 egg
- ➢ 1/4 cup fresh cream
- ➢ 1 tablespoon ghee
- ➢ Salt
- ➢ 2 cups spinach, boiled and blended
- ➢ 1/4 cup Parmesan cheese

DIRECTIONS:

1. Mix all the ingredients except the spinach.
2. Divide the dough and add the spinach to 2/3 of it.
3. In a small mold, put the green dough with a

teaspoon of white dough in the middle. Bake in the oven at 390° F (200° C) for 20 minutes.

NUTRITION:

Calories 598 Carbs 27g Fat 38g Protein 37g

8) Stuffed artichokes

INGREDIENTS:

- ➢ 4 artichokes
- ➢ 2 tablespoons Parmesan cheese
- ➢ 1/4 cup other soft cheese
- ➢ Parsley and chives
- ➢ Salt and pepper
- ➢ 1 egg
- ➢ 4 slices keto bread
- ➢ 1/2 cup almond milk
- ➢ 1 garlic clove
- ➢ Extra virgin olive oil to taste
- ➢ 2 ladles broth for stewing

DIRECTIONS:

1. Clean the artichokes, cut the bread into cubes and let it soften with the milk.
2. Add the grated cheeses, egg, salt, pepper and chopped herbs.
3. Mix and, once thick, fill the artichokes.
4. Fry a garlic clove in extra virgin olive oil, put the artichokes in the pan and add the broth.
5. Cover and cook over medium-low heat for 30/35 minutes.

NUTRITION:

Calories 596 Carbs 15g Fat 45g Protein 33g

59) Stuffed eggplants

INGREDIENTS:

- ➤ small eggplants
- ➤ 1 pound minced meat
- ➤ ripe tomatoes
- ➤ 2 eggs
- ➤ 3/4 cup Parmesan cheese
- ➤ Extra virgin olive oil to taste
- ➤ Salt and spices to taste

DIRECTIONS:

1. In a large pan with salted boiling water, blanch the eggplants cut in half for about 20 minutes. Drain the eggplants and let cool.
2. Once cold, remove the pulp and cut into cubes. Place the empty eggplants in a baking sheet and set aside.
3. In a deep pan, pour plenty of extra virgin olive oil, salt and spices to taste (for example garlic, parsley, mint, capers).
4. Fry the eggplant cubes, tomatoes and minced meat over low heat for about 15 minutes and let cool.
5. When completely cold, add to the mixture the previously beaten 2 eggs and the Parmesan cheese mixing well.
6. Now fill the eggplants and bake at 390° F (200° C) for 40 minutes.

NUTRITION:

Calories 1923 Carbs 82g Fat 109g Protein 155g

60) Stuffed zucchini

INGREDIENTS:

- ➤ 3 zucchinis
- ➤ 1 cup minced meat of your choice
- ➤ Garlic
- ➤ Oil
- ➤ Salt
- ➤ Chili pepper

DIRECTIONS:

1. Wash the zucchinis, cut them lengthwise and remove the pulp with a teaspoon.
2. Put the pulp in a pan with two tablespoons of extra virgin olive oil and two garlic cloves.
3. Allow to soften, remove the garlic, add salt and a little chili pepper to taste. Place in a bowl and combine with the minced meat.
4. Once you have obtained a homogeneous mixture, place it in the hollow created in the zucchinis.
5. Place the zucchinis in a baking sheet lightly greased with extra virgin olive oil, drizzle lightly and bake at 355° F (180° C) for about 30 minutes.

NUTRITION:

Calories 357 Carbs 22g Fat 4g Protein 59g

61) Sweet and sour red cabbage

INGREDIENTS:

- ➤ 1 1/2 pounds red cabbage
- ➤ 1 tablespoon apple cider vinegar
- ➤ 3 tablespoons olive oil
- ➤ Pink salt
- ➤ Pepper
- ➤ Cinnamon

DIRECTIONS:

1. Cut the red cabbage thinly.
2. In a nonstick pan, pour the oil and add the cabbage, salt and pepper, then the apple cider vinegar and cinnamon.
3. Stir and cover with a lid. Cook for 15 minutes

NUTRITION:

Calories 512 Carbs 21g Fat 43g Protein 11g

62) Zoodles with pesto, Parmesan cheese and almonds

INGREDIENTS:

- Zoodles (4 baby zucchinis)
- 2 tablespoons pesto
- 1/4 cup almonds
- 1/4 cup grated Parmesan cheese

DIRECTIONS:

1. In a blender place the almonds and Parmesan cheese and coarsely blend.
2. Transfer to a hot nonstick pan and stir to brown.
3. Serve on sautéed zoodles with pesto.

NUTRITION:

Calories 545 Carbs 35g Fat 33g Protein 27g

63) Zucchini and feta cheese soufflé

INGREDIENTS for about 12 soufflés:

For the dough:

- 4 eggs
- 1/4 cup milk
- 2 tablespoons grated Parmesan cheese
- 1 tablespoon fresh cream cheese (optional)
- 1 tablespoon olive oil
- Salt (optional, the feta is already salty)
- Pepper to taste
- Spices to taste (such as chives)

For the filling:

- 1 grated zucchini
- Greek feta cheese

DIRECTIONS:

1. Beat the eggs and add milk, cream cheese, Parmesan cheese and oil.
2. Fill the baking cups (or silicone molds) with the mixture and stuff with the grated zucchini and shredded feta.
3. Bake in the preheated oven at 355° F (180° C) for 35 minutes.
4. This dish can also be prepared the day before.

NUTRITION:

Calories 616 Carbs 11g Fat 47g Protein 38g

64) Zucchini, ham and mozzarella pancake

INGREDIENTS:

- 4 tablespoons almond flour
- 1 medium-sized zucchini
- 1/2 sachet baking powder
- 1 tablespoon coconut oil
- 2 tablespoons grana cheese
- 1 whole egg + 1 egg white
- Salt and pepper
- Cooked ham
- Mozzarella

DIRECTIONS:

1. Grate the zucchini, place it in a cloth and squeeze it as much as you can to remove all the water.
2. If necessary, do this 2 times.
3. Add the flour, eggs, oil, salt, pepper, grana cheese and baking powder.
4. Mix and pour the mixture in a lightly greased 5 inch pan.
5. Cook over low heat with the lid on for about 15 minutes. To check the cooking, do the toothpick test.
6. Take out the pancake, cut in half and stuff as you prefer, for example with ham and mozzarella. Heat for 1 minute in the microwave or in the air fryer.

NUTRITION:

Calories 807 Carbs 17g Fat 55g Protein 60g

65) Zucchini in sauce

INGREDIENTS:

- 5 ounces zucchini
- 2 tablespoons extra virgin olive oil
- 2 tablespoons apple cider vinegar
- Mint, parsley
- salt

DIRECTIONS:

1. Finely chop the zucchini.
2. Prepare the sauce with extra virgin olive oil, apple cider vinegar, mint, parsley and salt.
3. Pour everything over the zucchini. Prepare one day ahead and place in the fridge.

NUTRITION:

Calories 356 Carbs 7g Fat 36g Protein 1g

66) Zucchini noodle half-spheres

INGREDIENTS:

- 2 zucchinis
- 4 eggs
- 2 tablespoons Parmesan cheese, aged 36 months
- 1/2 cup liquid cream
- Salt pepper

DIRECTIONS:

1. Start by spiralizing the zucchinis and put them in a salad bowl with salt.
2. After 10 minutes, squeeze and put them in the silicone molds.
3. Beat the eggs with all the other ingredients and pour them over the zucchinis. Bake in the oven at 430° F (220° C) for 25/30 minutes.

NUTRITION:

Calories 495 Carbs 15g Fat 33g Protein 34g

67) Zucchini parmigiana

INGREDIENTS for 4 people:

- 3 cups zucchini
- 1 cup mozzarella cheese
- 1 cup grated grana cheese
- 3/4 cup cooked ham
- Salt to taste

DIRECTIONS:

1. Cut the zucchinis, grill them and salt them. Take a baking sheet and line it with baking paper.
2. Start layering the parmigiana, beginning with the zucchini and then gradually with the mozzarella, ham and grana cheese.
3. Bake at 355° F (180° C) until a golden crust has formed.

NUTRITION:

Calories 780 Carbs 16g Fat 50g Protein 68g

68) Zucchini rolls stuffed with shrimps and avocado

INGREDIENTS for 2 servings:

- 3 zucchinis
- 3 eggs
- 5 ounces cooked shrimps
- 1 avocado

DIRECTIONS:

1. Cut the zucchinis into slices lengthwise. Cook them with a drizzle of oil in the preheated oven at 390° F (200° C) for 5 minutes.
2. Add the beaten eggs and bake for another 5/7 minutes until golden brown.
3. Once taken out of the oven (be careful not to burn yourself!), spread the omelet on a flat surface and stuff with the avocado previously cut into cubes or thin slices and the shrimps.
4. Roll up and serve the roll cut into slices!

NUTRITION:

Calories 747 Carbs 21g Fat 46g Protein 62g

69) Zucchini soup en croute

INGREDIENTS:

- ➤ 2 zucchinis
- ➤ For the croute:
- ➤ 2 tablespoons ground sesame seeds
- ➤ 2 tablespoons ground linseeds
- ➤ 3/4 cup almond flour
- ➤ 2 tablespoons extra virgin olive oil
- ➤ 1/4 cup water
- ➤ Herb-flavored salt
- ➤ Hemp seeds (Sauton)
- ➤ Oregano

DIRECTIONS:

1. For the croute, mix the dry ingredients together, then add the water and make a compact dough.
2. Divide it in two and roll it out between 2 sheets of baking paper obtaining 2 discs. Bake them in the oven at 355° F (180° C) for 20 minutes and lay them upside down on a flat plate.
3. For the soup, sauté 2 zucchinis with herbs and ghee in a pan with a shallot.
4. Blend everything together and pour the mixture over the dough. You can enrich the soup with 1 tablespoon of hemp seeds.

NUTRITION:

Calories 783 Carbs30g Fat 63g Protein 24g

70) Zucchini spaghetti with bell pepper sauce

INGREDIENTS for 2 people:

- ➤ 2 zucchinis
- ➤ 1 red bell pepper
- ➤ 1 yellow bell pepper
- ➤ 1 green bell pepper
- ➤ 1 garlic clove
- ➤ 1 1/2 cups tomato puree
- ➤ 1 cup water
- ➤ 1 tablespoon extra virgin olive oil
- ➤ Salt to taste
- ➤ Pepper to taste
- ➤ Parsley to taste
- ➤ 1 sprinkle grated vegan cheese

DIRECTIONS:

1. To prepare the sauce, brown the previously chopped garlic clove in oil.
2. Cut the peppers as you like, cook them for a few minutes and add the tomato puree and water.
3. When the sauce is ready, add salt, pepper and parsley to taste.
4. At this point, cut the zucchinis into spaghetti with the appropriate tool.
5. Put them directly in the pan without blanching them in boiling water for a crispier texture and cook for 1/2 minute.
6. You can finish with a sprinkle of grated vegan cheese, for example Parmesan cheese.

NUTRITION:

Calories 363 Carbs 43g Fat 16g Protein 12g

WORKOUT

I will try to give you the basic principles of a proper training by providing you a specific 90-day training plan. Miracles just don't happen so easly, and no one can promise to have one (and be warned that nobody can promise it!).

Moreover, I really don't like to make fun of people, but I can guarantee you that by following this program your body and its performance will improve.

It's up to you to find out how much it could improve, since it depends on so many factors such as genetics, commitment, perseverance, food, etc.).

The first step to improve is to get starting this fitness program as soon as possible, avoiding any expression like: "I'll start on Monday!", you have to start right now!

I know that I'm not wrong by saying that 90% of women don't like their legs, they see them chubby and shapeless, or they think to have wide hips, a big butt or lots of cellulite, Those with legs that are too dry, those with a flat butt, etc., etc.. Very few people really like themselves!...Isn't it so?

It's not just related to female hormones, since it's too easy to only blame them and say there's nothing to be done about it!

Let's admit that women could have some disadvantage on that, but of course they can do it and never make up for it and improve their appearance.

Wrong supply food chain and non-existent training close the picture and lead you to the current state, which is why you started reading this article. If nowadays there is much more attention to what we eat, it is also beacause the increasingly hectic life forces us to incorrect habits, which affect our health and body and with a greater accumulation of fat in undesiderable places. Let's not talk about the workout that is the most lack between women...let's tell it like it is.... "You don't like to workout with what could be good for you: the weights!" We should disregard the way that loads fill you out and make you look manly... It's not like that, and I don't even want to waste time trying to convince you to follow this direction!

The only thing I can tell you is that weights can help you to get more toned and create those shapes you desire so much. But since women don't like weights and they don't like to workout with them, they always look for other ways to try to achieve their goal. That's why nowadays the industry that deals with female beauty is booming (especially in terms of turnover and incomes). [SEP] Be careful also to the weight loss centers, what they can do for you is only to make you lose some water, but that as soon as you get home you regain it by drinking!

However, how many people have started doing stupid exercises in those rooms heated to 50° where they spend and throw away a lot of money, because of clever sellers who just care to sell you the package of treatments, and do not care about anything else and use "dirty" psychological tricks, to convince you to buy them!

Be careful in this case too, you can lose <u>weight</u> (a lot of water, with the risk of dehydration and compromise your health) but you won't reach in any way the shape you want to. [SEP] A lot of people promise doing miracles, but as I mentioned before, nobody keeps their promise!

There are so many shortcuts that you can try nowadays and all with the same goal: certainly not your health, no one cares about you, the only thing they really care about is the money you can pay for it!

And once you paid, well perhaps you already know the story....

Let's leave the bad stuff alone and start talking seriously about how you can improve the appearance of your lower limbs. [SEP] A serious and well-planned workout is the only thing you need to improve your shape, creating that toned body you always desired to get.

The program that I want to set up for you, includes real exercises. I'm not talking of <u>press</u>, abductor, adductor, gluteus tool, and slings and slingers from the ground that you may know, but which also serve very little to shape your legs and your glutes. [SEP] If you <u>Personal Trainer</u> (for which you paid a lot I guess) provided you a sheet for lower limbs sheet similar to the following:

- Leg Press 3x15
- Abductor tool 3x15
- Adductor tool 3x15
- Gluteus tool 3x15

I highly recommend you to start thinking to change your PT.

It is not possible that a serious and well-qualified professional gave you these simple exercises without any committing on teaching you the fundamental exercises, technically difficult but that can do so much for your body.

You can undoubtedly do these activities all alone!

The tools are made specifically so that even inexperienced people can use them without getting hurt! These are the <u>fundamental exercises</u>, the ones you must learn to do to shape your body! But these exercises require a good trainer to teach you the correct gestures (just like the ski instructor teaches you how to ski!).

If athletes are choosing these tool-free exercises, there's probably more than one reason, right?

<u>Isotonic tools</u> are almost useless in physical training, except for a few pieces of equipment that can help you sometimes.

Here below the four exercises will shape your thighs and glutes:

- <u>Squat</u>
- <u>Forward Lunges</u>
- <u>Stretch legs</u>
- Step-up

There are other exercises as well, but these are enough to create a truly strong workout.

I'm not including photos or videos of these exercises, because if you're not familiar with them, it's best to have your trainer teach them to you the first time.

Try to find a really good and professional Personal Trainer in your area, subscribe few hours with him and let him teach you these exercises, these exercises are the foundation of any <u>legs workout</u>!

These exercises are technically difficult to do, which if not duly performed can cause damages. This is the reason why an initial period of adaptation is needed, especially to improve the technique of how to perform them. Avoid any training program that promises to let you reach super quick results in a very short time. In order to get some serious results you will need at least 90 days, just like the program that I want to share with you.

VOCABULARY USED: The first number represents how many SETS (or Series) and the second number how many REPS (or repetitions) for each Set. The Rest indicates when it's time to rest between each set.

Example: 4 (sets) x 12 (reps) - 60" rest. This means that you need to perform 12 reps 4 times resting 60 seconds between each time.

ECCENTRIC MOTION: Movement of only descent to the ground, without the push phase. The Eccentric reps are very slow and should be performed by descending with the seconds given to each sheet.

Please note: These Workouts are merely generic indications that do not consider all individual characteristics, such as any injuries, overweight, motor disability, etc...

1-4 weeks:	Adaptation Phase
Week 5-8:	Hypertrophic Phase
9-12week:	"Shaping" phase
Adaptation Phase 1-4 (4th week for discharge) *Days of training per week:* 3 of the duration of about 60 minutes *Method used:* repeated efforts	
Day 1	Warm-up 5'-10' jump rope Thighs-Glutes Squats_4x20; recovery between series 1'30" Stretch Legs_4x20; recovery between series 1'30" Forward Lunges 3x15 for each side; recovery between series 1'30" Abdomen 2 exercises of your choice Cool-down 10' of stretching
Day 2	Choose a program for the top part of your body
Day 3	Warm-up 5'-10' jump rope Thighs-Glutes Squat 4x20; recovery between sets 1'30 " Stretch legs 4x20; recovery between sets 1'30" Step-up 3x15 for each side; recovery between sets 1'30" Abdomen 2 exercises of your choice Cool-down 10' of stretching
Hypertrophy phase 5-8 (4th week for discharge) *Days of training per week:* 3 of the duration of about 60 minutes *Method used:* Superseries	
Day 1	Warm-up 5'-10' jump rope Thighs-Buttocks

	Squat in <u>Superset</u> with Step-up (8+8)x5; recovery 2 minutes after the second exercise Superset Stretch legs with Forward Lunges (8+8)x5; recovery 2 minutes after the second exercise Abdomen 2 exercises of your choice Cool-down 10' of stretching
Day 2	Choose a program for the top part of your body
Day 3	Warm-up 5'-10' jump rope Thighs-Glutes Squat in Superset with Step-up (8+8)x5; recovery 2 minutes after the second exercise Superset Stretch legs with Forward Lunges (8+8)x5; recovery 2 minutes after the second exercise Abdomen 2 exercises of your choice Cool-down 10' of stretching

Phase of "Shaping" 9-12 (4th week for discharge) *Days of training per week:* 3 of the duration of about 60 minutes *Method used:* Superseries - complete in the shortest time possible the proposed work, recovery time depends on you, use the time to recovery while moving with one station then onto the next to finish the following series.	
Day 1	Warm-up 5'-10' jump rope Thighs-Glutes Squats in Superset with Step-up (6+6)x10; recovery between exercises is subjective, the minimum necessary. Superset Stretch legs with Forward Lunges (6+6)x10; recovery between exercises is subjective, the minimum necessary. Abdomen 2 exercises of your choice Cool-down 10' of stretching
Day 2	Choose a program for the top part of your body
Day 3	Warm-up 5'-10' jump rope Thighs-Glutes Squat in Superset with Stretch legs (6+6)x10; recovery between exercises is subjective, the minimum necessary. Step-up in Superset with Forward Lunges (6+6)x10; recovery between exercises is subjective, the minimum necessary. Abdomen 2 exercises of your choice Cool-down 10' of stretching

Here your schedule!

You have 90 days to give the best of yourself and get the results you've been looking for.

The program is very strong, it implies a lot of sacrifices (health food balance and a good lifestyle) but it will also give you a lot of satisfaction.

If you don't believe it, you can take a picture of you before starting the program and a picture at the end of the 90 days, compare them to check on any kind of improvement on your body.

Do it!!! It will help you take what you are doing seriously and reach your goal. This is all you need to do to improve your legs and glutes: a good workout program. Disregard easy routes, it is just a misuse of your valuable time and cash.

Good training, good nutrition and an excellent lifestyle is the winning recipe for your legs and glutes.

For those who do not have time to go to the gym, here is a list of simple exercises, from which you can pick and choose 4 or 5 to perform in the comfort of your own home.

Clearly, not using any overloads (as for training in the gym) is difficult and pretty much impossible to set a progression of load ... however you can still increase the series and reducing the reps in the first 3 weeks and do a week of discharge (the fourth one), and then start the cycle of 4 weeks in the fifth week, and so on for 12 weeks.

Here's an example:

Week 1: Squat 3x 12; Back Squat 3x12 Front Squat 3x12 ....and so on, by following the exercises explained below

Week 2: Squat 4x9 ; Back Squat 4x9 Front Squat 4x9 .... and so on, by following the exercises explained below

Week 3: 5 x 6; Squat 5x6 ; Back squat 5x6 Front squat 5x6 .... and so on, by following the exercises explained below

Week 4: 2x15; Squat 12 x15 ; Back squat 2x15 Front squat 2x15 .... and so on, by following the exercises explained below

Week 5: Same as week 1 and so on.,..

The recoveries between each series will be a little lower (between 45 and 60 seconds)

The first improvements should be seen after just a couple of months, but when it comes to B-side training, the key is to keep the rhythm up. If you're wishing to wear a skinny jeans, the main advice to give you is to make this workout part of your weekly fitness routine, preceded by a brief 10-minute of cardio warm-up and followed by some stretching exercises.

Standing exercises

Squat

A primary glute workout exercise, it is performed by starting with your feet perpendicular to your shoulders. From that position, kneel down, expanding your arms out in front and pushing your butt back as though you are going to sit in a chair. Then stop when your thighs are lined up to the ground and carry your weight to your heels.

Back Squat

This exercise primarily develops the external muscle of the glute.

Position yourself as if you were going to perform a normal squat. Bend your knees bringing your right leg back and when your left thigh is parallel to the ground, push up with your left heel and return to the beginning position.

Front Squat

With your hands on your waist, step forward and bend your knee, leaving the opposite leg extended back. Then stop when your thigh is lined up with the ground and return to the beginning position.

Broad jump

Keep your legs matching your shoulder width and place your arms along your sides. Squat down and jump as far as you can, utilizing your arms to impel yourself forward. Land on your forefeet, promptly hunch down and jump once more.

Plié squat

A merge between fitness and dance, this sequence works the inner thighs as well as the glutes.

With hands on waist, legs apart and feet turned outward, bend knees, squatting as much as possible. Return to an upright position pushing up with your heels and squeezing inner thighs and glutes.

Side lunge

Develops the sides of the glutes and inner and outer thighs.

Feet together, move one sideways by bending the corresponding knee and keeping the opposite leg extended and still. Return to beginning position.

Squat pulses

With your feet perpendicular to shoulder width and your hands clasped, squat down but instead of getting fully up, stop at half height and come down again.

Floor exercises

Backward leg lift

Lie face down, resting your face on your arms folded on the floor.

Lift one leg, bringing it up as high as possible and keeping the ankle soft.

Leg kickbacks

Stand on all fours and with your ankle bent, extend your right leg back until it is parallel to the ground.

At the moment of maximum extension tighten the glutes and return to the beginning position.

Superman

Lie face down on the floor with your arms forward and legs broadened.

Lift chest and legs as high as possible while keeping neck stiff.

Bridge

Lie supine with your knees twisted and your arms down the sides with your palms on the ground.

Push the heels together, lift up shaping a straight line between your chest area and knees. Squeeze your glutes together before returning to the beginning position.

Clamshell

This exercise works primarily on the gluteus medius.

Lie on your side with knees bent, legs on top of each other, one hand on your side and one supporting your head, arm bent. Without detaching your heels from each other, lift your outside leg as high as possible and gradually take it back to the beginning position.

Plank upwards

Sit on the floor with your legs extended, your back slightly bent back, and your arms straight with your palms on the floor.

Lift yourself up so your body frames a straight line from head to toe. Hold the position for about 10–15 seconds.

For lazy people, here are some exercises you can do at home with a towel.

Even if until now you have always seen the towels or kitchen towels useful for doing other things in your daily life, such as dusting or wiping sweat, hands and the rest of the body, you will soon discover that you can also perform many fitness exercises.

Towels can be used for:

- tone and strengthen the muscles of the whole body;
- train the cardiovascular system;
- improve muscle and joint flexibility.

The towels, thanks to their versatility, can be used to slide on the floor with hands and feet, to give tension, to perform displacements, to facilitate muscle stretches etc....

How to choose the right towel or rag

Almost all towels and rags slide across the floor, but it may happen that a floor has special joints and shapes that prevent smooth sliding. If you can't get a smooth glide you can use couch cushions, which allow for unrestrained sliding. Whether or not, you can wear shoes depends on you and according to the type of exercise you need to perform.

If you have big enough socks, you can try doing the gliding exercises directly with the socks, without shoes or towel and rags.

If you want a more professional tool, instead of a rag, at a very low cost ranging from $6 to $10, you can purchase fitness sliders.

We offer you 10 towel-exercises and 2 stretching exercises to add to your workout routine.

Plank upwards with side leg raise

Assume a plank position on your hands and place a towel under your right foot. Remain stable in your plank position and activate your core. Keep your legs overstretched and slide your right leg aside. Do not move your hips as you slide your right leg to the side. Then slide again and return to the plank position. Complete 10-15 reps with the right leg and then switch to the other leg.

Plank upwards spiderman with push up

Assume a plank position on your hands and place a towel under each foot. Stay stable in your plank position and activate your core. Starting with your legs straight, slide your right leg forward as if to touch your right arm and then your left leg. Then return to your plank position and immediately perform an arm bend. Do not move your hips as you slide your left and right leg forward. Complete 10 reps with the right leg and 10 with the left leg alternately and 10 push ups.

Back lunge

Start standing and transfer your weight slowly to your left leg, while placing a towel under your right foot. Slightly extend your right foot behind you, and stay with just your toes resting on the towel. Lower into a lunging position with your left leg, twisting your left knee at a 90-degree point and keeping your knee over your lower leg. As you lower yourself, slide your right foot behind you. Press down on your left heel to active your glutes and the muscles at the back of your thigh, straighten your left leg and return forward with your right leg. Repeat 15-20 times with the right leg and then switch legs.

Side lunge

Start standing, move your weight gradually to your left leg and keep your right foot into the towel. Lower your left leg into a 90-degree side lunge position and slide your right leg to the side. Use the glutes and the hind muscles of the left leg to go up, while using the inner thigh of the right leg to slide the right foot back and forth to the side. Carry out15-20 reps on each side.

Hamstring twists

Lie down in supine position. Keep your knees twisted and your feet laying on the floor in a bridge position. Put a towel under each foot and raise your hips by forming a bridge. Keep your glutes and back thigh muscles active as you slide your feet forward until your legs are almost straight and stay with your hips lifted. Use your back thigh muscles to press into the floor and slide your feet back into the bridge position. Carry out 15-20 reps without allowing your hips to drop to the ground.

Hikers

Begin in an upwards board position with a towel under each foot. Keep your core tight and spine in a neutral position as you pull your knees toward your chest and extend your leg back as if to simulate a horizontal climb. Utilize your glutes and hamstrings to stretch your thigh and your abs to pull your knees toward your chest. Alternate sides as quickly as possible and repeat from 30 seconds to one minute.

Sliding triangle

Start in an upwards plank position resting on your hands with a towel under both toes. Keep your legs straight and pull both legs apart, sliding your feet inward, more or less in the center, which is represented by the distance between your hands and feet from your starting point. You should find yourself with your hips up in an almost triangle position, where your hands and feet are the base. Active your abs to raise and lower your hips. Don't let your hips fall down with your lower back and stay with your legs straight. Complete 10-15 reps.

Upward plank with leg circumduction

Expect the position of plank on your hands and put a towel under each foot. Stay stable in your plank position and activate your core. Slide the towels and feet as if to draw a circle, then bend and extend your legs as you draw the circle. Do not move your hips as you slide and rotate your legs. Complete 10 circles with your right leg and 10 with your left leg.

Push up on the side

Start in an upwards plank position with a towel placed under each hand. As you lower yourself down twist your left arm into a push-up, push your right arm aside. Push up, extend your left arm again as you slide your right arm back into the beginning position. Complete 5-10 reps and then switch sides.

V sit up

Sit on an exercise mat and hold the ends of a towel between your hands. Bend and lift your legs so that your shins are almost parallel to the floor. Shift your bust back slightly to balance your weight on your tailbone. Hold the towel in front of you, active your core, pull your knees toward your chest and bring the towel toward your shins. Pull your knees away from your chest almost to the point of extending your legs and lift the towel with your arms straight above your head. Repeat for 10 times.

Stretching

Towels can also be very useful for stretching, both at the end of your workout and for your daily routine: remember that stretching always brings significant benefits.

Back extension

Lie on your stomach and spot a towel under each hand as you expand your arms out before you. Active your core, extend your spine and make your hands slide towards you while lifting your chest and shoulders off the floor. Make sure you don't feel any compression in your spine; you don't want to lift too high. Stay a few seconds and then slide back down. Repeat 10-15 times.

Leg extension

Lay down on your back with your legs stretched out. Raise your right leg and spot the towel under the sole of the foot. Pull your toes down fully extend your leg and stay for 30 seconds. Repeat with the left leg.

How to perform the exercises

You can perform each exercise for 2 or 3 sets. If while performing the exercises you feel tired and you are not able to complete the required number of reps in a row, take a small break and then start again until you complete the repetition.

Now let's see how to set up a perfect workout to train your chest and arm.

First thing, you need to identify how many time per week you need to train.

- Usually the number of times is 3, because 3 is the perfect number in training; however, if we want to better focus our concentration on the muscular work we are doing, perhaps it is better to train an extra day, reducing the exercises and the time of each session.

- So in this case we recommend 4 sessions per week.

The exercises in this case should not exceed 60 minutes of total work, we must be full of energy, determined and focused from the first very minute of our training session until the last one.

Long sessions lead to an expenditure of physical and mental energy that with a 4-day

splite routine is disruptive.

TRAINING CARD

DAY 1 - PECS & TRICEPS

1. **Flat Bench Press with Handlebars** 2 Rounds of 8 Reps (that's only 2 sets taken to muscle failure)
2. **Flat Bench Low Cables Fly** 2 Rounds of 12 Reps
3. **Incline Bench Press with Barbell with Grip and Elbows Stretched** 2 Rounds of 8 Reps
4. **Handlebar Crunches on Incline Bench** 2 Rounds of 12 Reps
5. **Parallel Dip or Rings** 1 round to muscle failure (max number of reps)
6. **Extensions behind the neck with rope on low cable** 2 Rounds of 12 Reps
7. **One-Handed High Cable Push Down** 1-2 rounds of 12 reps

DAY 2 - LATS & BICEPS

1. **Lat Equipment pulldown Chest 2** Rounds of 8 Reps (that's just 2 sets taken to muscle failure)
2. **Handlebars Pullover** 2 Rounds of 12 Reps
3. **Bust flexed rower with 2 Handlebars** 2 rounds of 8 reps
4. **Pulley** 2 Rounds of 12 Reps
5. **Bar tractions reverse grip and tight** 1 round to muscle failure (max number of reps)
6. **Curl with Handlebars on Incline Bench** 2 Rounds of 12 Reps
7. **Concentration Handlebars Curl** 1-2 Rounds of 12 reps

DAY 3 - REST

DAY 4 - LEGS

1. **Deadlift** 2 Rounds of 8 Reps (that's just 2 sets taken to muscle failure)

2. **Front Squat** 2 Rounds of 8 Reps

3. **45° Press** 2 Rounds of 8 Reps

4. **Leg Curl** 2 Rounds of 12 Reps

5. **Leg Extension** 2 rounds of 12 reps

6. <u>**Standing Calf**</u> 2 rounds of 20 reps

7. **Calf on Press or Seated Calf or Donkey Calf** 2 rounds of 20 reps

DAY 5 - SHOULDERS - TRAPS and ABDOMINALS

1. **Seated Slow Forward** 2 rounds of 8 Reps (that's just 2 sets taken to muscle failure)

2. **Side push-up with handlebars on incline bench** 2 Series of 12 reps machinper arm

3. <u>**90° Raises**</u> **with handlebars with the head supported on the bench** 2 rounds of 12   reps

4. **Handlebar shrugs with bust supported on incline bench** 2 rounds of 12 reps

5. **Chin pulls with** <u>**barbell ez**</u> 2 rounds of 12 reps

6. **Knees to chest hanging on the bar** 2 rounds of 12 reps

7. **Abdominal tool** 2 rounds of 12 reps

8. **Crunch for obliques on the ground** 2 rounds of 12 reps per side

Remarks: Keep recovery time to minimum, and try to set your recovery on one minute between each set.

CHEST TRAINING FOR BEGINNERS

If you are starting from the beginning, start with these training sheets in order to begin developing Pectorals and Triceps as correctly, gradually and effectively as possible. Start with training 1 and move on to the next ones only when you reach the final requirement of each training.

Training 1

- Knee push-ups: 4 x Max, 60sec rest between sets
- Squat Knees: 4 x Max, 90sec rest between sets
- Eccentric Squats (only slow descent): 4 Eccentrics in 6 seconds, 20sec rest between the Eccentrics

When you get to 4×6 in Knee push-ups, move on to the next Card.

Training 2

- Classic push-ups: 4 x 2-4, 120sec rest between sets
- Knee push-ups: 4 x 6-8, 60sec rest between sets

When you get to do 6 complete Classic push-ups in a row, move on to the next Card.

Training 3

- Classic squats: 4 x 6-8, 90sec rest between sets
- Tight Squats: 4 x 4, 60sec rest between sets
- Knee push-ups: 2 x Max, 90sec rest between sets

When you get to 8 Classic push-ups for 3-4 sets, switch to the full Premium Program

Training **1**

- Chest press: 4 x 12, 75sec rest between sets
- Knee push-ups: 4 x Max, 75sec rest between sets
- Eccentric Squats (slow descent only): 4 Eccentrics in 6 seconds, 20sec rest between Eccentrics

When you get to 4×6 in Knee push-ups, move on to the next Card.

Training 2

- Bench: 4 x 8-10-12-15, 90sec rest between sets
- Crisscross cables: 4 x 8, 60sec rest between sets
- Knee push-ups: 4 x Max, 60sec rest between sets

Printed in Great Britain
by Amazon

15940921R00086